Demystifying the
Nurse/Therapist Consultant

Published in 2005 by:
Nelson Thornes Ltd
Delta Place
27 Bath Road
CHELTENHAM
GL53 7TH
United Kingdom

05 06 07 08 09 10/ 10 9 8 7 6 5 4 3 2 1

A catalogue record for this book is available from the British Library

ISBN 0 7487 8089 0

Illustrations by Clinton Banbury
Page make-up by Northern Phototypesetting Co. Ltd

Printed and bound in Spain by GraphyCems

Acknowledgements

Opening quotation from *To Kill a Mockingbird* by Harper Lee copyright © 1960
by Harper Lee. Renewed copyright © 1988 by Harper Lee. Foreword
copyright © 1993 by Harper Lee. Reprinted by permission of HarperCollins
Publishers Inc.
Figure 2.4 'Illustrations of formal organisational relationships' from
Management and Organisational Behaviour sixth edition by Laurie J Mullins,
Pearson Education Ltd copyright © Laurie J Mullins 2002.
Figure 4.3 'Raising awareness and the profile of the NTC' copyright © Crown
copyright. Crown copyright material is reproduced with the permission of the
Controller of the HMSO and the Queen's Printer for Scotland.
Figure 4.5 'Framework for highly effective people' taken from *The 7 Habits of
Highly Effective People* by Stephen R Covey (1989) Simon and Schuster, New
York.
Figure 5.2 from *Consultant Nursing in Mental Health* copyright © 2005 Gary
Wilshaw used by permission of Kingsham Press, Chichester.
Figure 5.3 from *Consultant Nursing in Mental Health* copyright © 2005 Gary
Wilshaw used by permission of Kingsham Press, Chichester.
Figure 6.6 'Sickness care model versus chronic care model' copyright ©
Crown copyright. Crown copyright is reproduced with the permission of the
Controller of the HMSO and the Queen's Printer for Scotland.

Every effort has been made to contact the copyright holders but if any have
been inadvertently overlooked, the publishers will be pleased to make the
necessary arrangement at the first opportunity.

Demystifying the Nurse/Therapist Consultant

A Foundation Text

Rob McSherry and Sarah Johnson (eds)

CONTENTS

Atticus was right. One time he said you never really know a man until you stand in his shoes and walk around in them.

Harper Lee, *To Kill a Mockingbird*

PREFACE

The health and social care sector of the United Kingdom is a large and complex body, with National Health Service spending currently estimated at £50 billion per annum. It is forecast that this will rise to £76 billion by 2005/06, with a steady growth in the workforce of 1% per annum. This trend of rising costs and an increasing number of personnel is set to continue, and with it comes a recognition that an appropriate skill mix is required in the workforce to deliver a high-quality service (Department of Health, 2003b).

The NHS Plan (Department of Health, 2000) stated for the first time that nurses and other staff would have the opportunity to extend their roles. The introduction of the Nurse/Therapist Consultant (NTC) post is an integral part of this commitment to modernisation, its aim being to enable advanced clinical practitioners to influence decision-making at a strategic level while maintaining patient contact (NHS Executive, 1999).

We use the term 'Nurse/Therapist Consultant' in its broadest sense; 'nurse', for example, represents nurses, midwives and health visitors, whereas 'therapist' represents those clinical professionals termed the 'allied health professions'. With the implementation of the *Agenda for Change* (DoH, 2003a), all these professions will have consultant posts identified within their career pathways in the near future. The NTC role has the potential to be both exciting and challenging for the individual, the service and the professions. Preliminary targets for 2004 were set at 1000 posts for nurses and 250 for the allied health professionals (NHS Executive, 1999). The four key components of these posts have been identified as:

- enhancing the career structure and opportunities for experienced and expert staff wishing to remain in clinical practice
- leading and developing changes in practice for improved patient outcomes
- developing educational and training opportunities for clinical staff
- leading research at a strategic and local level.

There are currently fewer people in post than anticipated, figures of 800 Nurse and 30 Therapist Consultants having recently been quoted (DoH, 2002). The reasons for this may include a lack of a coherent staff development strategy, professional and interprofessional funding concerns, and health professionals themselves being uncertain about meeting the requirements for these complex posts.

It is hoped that health and social care professionals will, through this book, develop a clearer understanding of the NTC role and feel confident to apply for these new, very exciting posts.

The editors would like to acknowledge that although this text predominately refers to NTCs in England, the principles may be transferred to NTCs in the other home countries of the United Kingdom.

Rob McSherry, Sarah Johnson
2004

REFERENCES

Department of Health (2000) *The NHS Plan: A Plan for Investment, a Plan for Reform.* HMSO, London.

Department of Health (2002) *NHS Hospital and Community Health Services Non-Medical Workforce Census England.* DoH, Leeds.

Department of Health (2003a) *Agenda for Change – proposed agreement.* HMSO, London.

Department of Health (2003b) *Health Sector Workforce Market Assessment.* Skills For Health, London.

National Health Service Executive (1999) *Health Service Circular 1999/217 Nurse, midwifery, and health visitor consultant: Establishing posts and making appointments.* NHS Executive, London.

1 THE CONTEXT OF THE MODERNISATION AGENDA

Rob McSherry, Margaret Murray and Sarah Johnson

INTRODUCTION

The National Health Service (NHS) employs over 2 million people across a wide range of occupations, over 400,000 of whom (including nurses, midwives and health visitors) are registered via a nursing professional body, more than 66,000 being registered as allied health professionals (AHPs) (Department of Health, 2003b). This large organisation has been the subject of reform and modernisation in order to meet the demands of the twenty-first century. In 1997, *The New NHS – Modern, Dependable* (DoH, 1997) looked at reconfiguring the workforce to reduce demarcation between professional roles and to clearly identify standards, accountability and evidence-based practice (Wilson-Barnett, 2003).

This was followed up by *The NHS Plan* (DoH, 2000), which described new ways of working to improve patient care and make the best use of a skilled workforce within finite resources. It was also envisaged that this would help to increase staff numbers as it would ensure greater job satisfaction across the workforce.

In a speech to the Nurse '98 awards, the Prime Minister announced the introduction of Nurse Consultants. This was followed up by a commitment to establishing the role in the national strategy documents *Making a Difference* (DoH, 1999) for the nursing professions and *Meeting the Challenge* (2000) for the allied health professions.

The introduction of the Nurse/Therapist Consultant (NTC) is said to be 'ground-breaking' as it recognises the full contribution of these professions in the health and social care arena (DoH, 2002). Averil Imison, Head of Policy for AHPs at the Department of Health, said in 2002:

> It is important that people can see that they are being taken seriously as director or management material or in their clinical role. If the top ten to twenty per cent of the professions see themselves as potential directors or consultants it will make a huge difference in encouraging people to stay in the NHS.

The Changing Workforce Programme was set up to help with managing the changes. This included looking at the allocation of responsibilities across clinical specialities, expanding the breadth and depth of current jobs and designing and implementing new ones. In diabetes care, for example, the advanced clinical skills of Nurse Consultants may mean that they see the patients with the more complex problems; similarly, in dietetics, the AHP Consultant may work with medical and nursing colleagues to draw up care and referral protocols for patients (Hargadon, 2001; British Dietetic Association, 2002).

Dowling et al (1996) felt that the implementation of the European Working Time Directive, leading to a reduction in the number of junior doctors' hours, might have resulted in the government having to identify different ways and patterns of working and also influenced the development of new posts. Some may see the introduction of the NTC as a challenge as they interpret it as a way of covering up recruitment shortages and gaps in specialist knowledge or practice, therefore viewing its introduction with some suspicion. The Department of Health (1999) suggests that the establishment of the NTC posts will:

> Help to provide better outcomes for patients by improving services and quality, strengthening clinical leadership and providing new career opportunities in order to retain expert nurse/therapists.

From this, it would appear that a number of issues have led to the development of these posts:

- the modernisation agenda, which encourages the development of services based around patients' needs
- redesigning the role and structure of leadership within interdisciplinary teams and services
- the recruitment, training and retention of expert clinical staff in practice
- the move from specialist to expert consultant practice
- embedding a culture of evidence-based practice and lifelong learning within the workforce (DoH, 2003b; DoH, 2003a).

Drivers for the NTC within the National Health Service

Activity 1.1   *Reflective question* _____

Identifying the drivers for the NTC

What factors do you feel have led to the introduction of NTC posts?

Read on and compare your findings with those in the Activity Feedback at the end of this section.

In Activity 1.1, you should have identified that the primary origins of these factors can be traced back to a combination of societal changes associated with rising public expectations (DoH, 1992). The media continues to report major clinical incidents and declines in the standard of services within the NHS (Smith, 1998). Wilkinson and Miers (1999) discuss the public's lack of confidence in the NHS and believe that it could be attributed to insufficient investment, poor management or unsuccessful government reform. This has been further compounded by a number of serious clinical incidents that have added to the public's unease and led them to believe that the overall standards and quality of service are poor throughout the United Kingdom (McSherry and Haddock, 1999).

The impact of *The Citizens Charter* (DoH, 1993) and *The Patient's Charter* (DoH, 1992) was seen to be effective because both public and health care professionals became better informed. The public has also become more interested in health- and policy-related issues (Shuttleworth, 1992; Morris and Herriot 1994; Royal College of Nursing, 1994), which is still the case today. As a result, patients and their families are not prepared to accept lower standards of practice but try to seek satisfactory outcomes through the courts (Wilson, 1996). Over the past decade, there has been an increase in the number of formal complaints made by patients and carers about hospital and community services. Some of these have led to litigation, the estimated cost of clinical negligence for 2000/01 being £500 million (Wilson and Tingle, 1999).

The aim is to have a blame-free culture that encourages members of staff openly to report, discuss and learn from any clinical incidents or complaints that may arise. These may be procedural failures rather than individuals' actions or omissions. Training and education should aim to make health care professionals aware of this situation so that they will develop the competence and confidence to deal positively with difficult situations. Complaints can be reduced by ensuring that the information communicated to patients/carers is relevant to them and based upon the best available evidence. Hopefully, the development of evidence-based practice will enhance communication and reduce the number of complaints (Browne, 1996).

Advances in technology, particularly the Internet, have given the public easier access to information. Only a few years ago, much of this information would have been difficult to obtain, but it is now driving patients' and families' expectations. Technology has led to the development of new equipment that enables the quality and the standards of health care to be enhanced. Pressure-relieving devices and computerised moving and handling equipment are examples of this developing technology. All have the potential to enhance the quality of care delivered by health care professionals in practice.

It is important, as Dineen and Walshe (1999) point out, that the service is confident that staff have the appropriate knowledge, competence and skills to use such equipment safely. Difficulties may arise when time and resources have to be set aside for the education and training of staff within the busy clinical environment. The added stress of balancing efficiency and effectiveness within the workplace while learning new skills will be considerable as staff will be keen to maintain high-quality standards in their patient care. The aspirations of patients and their families for improved care delivery cannot be achieved unless new systems are also developed; these will need government backing and adequate resourcing.

A major concern is the rising number of patients admitted to hospital with multiple and complex needs; health care providers have had to change their patterns of health care delivery to accommodate this group. In some areas, acute medical or surgical assessment units have been introduced to maximise the use of acute and community beds and encourage collaborative working between primary and secondary care. Public and private sector partnerships are becoming increasingly common. For example, an acute illness may be initially treated in hospital, with a longer period of rehabilitation undertaken in a private nursing home. The problem of 'bed-blocking', as the media has called it, has been addressed through the introduction of 'hospital at home' schemes; these enable individuals to return home supported by experienced health and care staff.

In conclusion, NTCs seem to be in an ideal position to facilitate and support the delivery of the government's reforms as they have a strategic overview and are able to look at the wider picture. The challenge will be to place this role at an appropriate level that will both initiate and direct service developments while obtaining acceptance from all members of the team and professional hierarchy.

Activity 1.1   *Feedback* _____

Identifying the drivers for the NTC

A combination of societal, political and professional factors have contributed to the introduction of NTC posts:
- the government's modernisation reforms, leading to changes in the way in which health care is organised and delivered
- a lack of confidence in the NHS owing to perceived poor standards and low quality of practice
- the threat of litigious action
- technological advances
- accommodating the reduction in junior doctors' hours resulting from changes in the European Working Time Directives
- recruitment and retention issues for nurses and therapists
- the career structure of nurses and therapists in clinical practice.

IDENTIFYING AND DEVELOPING THE NTC ROLE

A central challenge for the NTC is one of status. The true measure of the role will be in demonstrating the achievement of independent and autonomous practice. Becoming 'autonomous' (having the power or right to self-govern without interference from other professions or administrative forces) requires the NTC to have the freedom and authority to act independently (Kelly and Joet, 1995; Creasia and Parker, 1996), 'independence' in this instance referring to the ability to direct practice.

NTC posts are not meant to substitute for those of junior doctors but are instead a new way of working to achieve modernisation (Jones, 2002). The intention is to challenge and embrace new and existing ways of working, the emphasis being on the extension of professional boundaries. Success will be measured by whether they provide an efficient and effective service that meets patients' needs (Wilson-Barnet 2003).

The key roles of the NTC will enable the interprofessional team to work effectively and ensure that the services developed hold the patient at the centre of their concerns. It is envisaged that this approach will replace the traditional hierarchies often seen within health care and help to deliver the government's modernisation agenda. NTCs should have the freedom to function independently, with support from peers and management and with adequate resources to work effectively within an open organisational culture (O'Gardy, 1986, cited in Creasia and Parker, 1996).

Some posts are linked to target-specific health inequalities or aim to improve access to services (DoH, 2000). The Chartered Society of Physio-therapy (2002) has stated that the establishment of NTC posts is directly related to national initiatives and current government priorities and targets, including:

- cutting waiting lists and times
- tackling coronary heart disease, cancer and mental health
- handling emergencies more effectively
- strengthening primary care
- improving services for older people
- strengthening the front line.

This will lead to the development of a range of services that reflect local need and community concerns.

IMPLEMENTING AND EVALUATING THE NTC ROLE

NTCs will play an important role within the government's modernisation programme as new and creative ways of working are developed. They will be able to make lasting changes to practice through collaborative working, building partnerships and improving access to information and networks (Manley, 2001). The four key functions of the role (expert practice, leadership, education and research) will be evident in all job descriptions. These may be linked directly to clinical pathways such as stroke, cancer and mental health, or more widely to an area of practice such as accident and emergency care. Bernadette Porter, a Nurse Consultant for multiple sclerosis, sees her role as one that influences decision-making at the highest level:

> We have developed integrated care pathways introducing nurse led clinics that ensure continuity of care with a named nurse. We have also recently won a research grant that allows us to complete a project looking at where is the best place for patients to have intravenous treatment for relapses, as an outpatient or in their own home?

As services are changing, new networks are being established. For example, the Nurse Consultant Network for nurses working in older people services and intermediate care has been meeting regularly for over a year and is acknowledged by members to be proving a valuable exchange of information between the field and policy (NHS, 2003).

The implementation of a new role will require evaluation (McSherry and Bassett, 2002). As these new posts are developmental, they will require evaluation in order to justify their cost and status (Pilling, 2003) and was seen as part of a service evaluation (Greenough et al, 1997). A previous analysis of expertise in nursing has led to a number of criteria being identified that are deemed 'expert'; these include peer recognition, experience, educational attainment, personal qualities, professional activities and status (Wilson-Barnett, 2003).

Benner's (1984) work, looking at the development from novice to expert, led her to identify some expert attributes that require advanced thinking and practice. She describes the ability to look at the wider picture and to take into account the complexities of the patient's life – as all are individual and unique. These may be features that NTCs will build into their self-evaluation, and the team may then be able to compare these with their own perceptions to gather evidence to support developments within the role. As the posts are still very new, evaluation methods have largely grown in a rather ad hoc local fashion, which will undoubtedly have to change. These are important and expensive posts and must therefore be seen to give value for money as well as providing a strategic lead in clinical services.

NURSE/THERAPIST SPECIALIST VERSUS NTC

So what are the differences between the roles and responsibilities of Nurse/Therapist Specialists and NTCs?

Activity 1.2   Reflective question _____

Identifying the differences between Nurse/Therapist Specialists and NTCs

Write down the differences between Nurse/Therapist Specialists and NTCs.
Read on and compare your findings with those in the Activity Feedback at the end of this section.

Some of the challenges facing the NTC will be:

- defining the role and responsibilities of the post
- identifying the personal skills and attributes necessary for the post
- developing the ability to discriminate between specialist and consultant practice.

Richley (2000), Adams et al (1997) and Sidani and Irvine (1999) outline the distinguishing features of the Specialist and Consultant roles. Looking at and summarising Table 1.1, it would appear that the specialist role can be defined as an expert role focused on a particular patient group that is Nurse/Therapist led, clinic based and case specific with a remit to improve the patient's quality of life, health or well-being, whereas the NTC demonstrates leadership at a strategic level within a clinical speciality through advancing and evaluating practice. The role is autonomous and independently managed.

Table 1.1 Comparing and contrasting the Nurse/Therapist Specialist and NTC roles

Specialist	Consultant
Diagnostic, has caseload expertise, advanced practitioner	Clinical specialist, expert practitioner
Clinical leader and/or manager in specific practice area	Clinical leader responsible for developing strategy and practice across a clinical speciality or service
Clinic led – actively involved in the interdisciplinary team, patient based working with family and carers	Clinical advisor with complex cross-boundary and interagency working
Utilises evidence-based practice and contributes to research within practice	Leads research and development, develops education and training opportunities
Ability to manage change	Leads and develop changes in practice to promote excellence

Recent literature associated with the Specialist and Consultant roles (Adams et al, 1997; Nurse Practitioner UK, 1999; Sneed, 1991; Wilson-Barnett, 2003) has identified some issues that are emerging for the NTC in the future (Figure 1.1). These are outlined below.

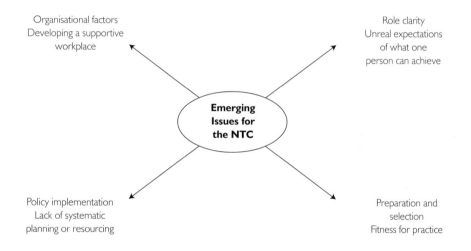

Figure 1.1 Emerging issues for the NTC

Role clarity, unreal expectations of what one person can achieve

The *Agenda for Change* (DoH, 2003a) will provide a clear career structure, NTCs being at the top of the 'skills escalator'. These new posts carry with them rather weighty expectations as the health professions have been waiting for recognition at this level for many years. This carries a great responsibility for individual NTCs, who may find the unreal expectations of others difficult to match. It will be important to establish a framework of competencies that enable all to understand this new role realistically so that NTCs will feel confident and competent within the post.

Preparation and selection, fitness for practice

The Health Service Circular 217 (DoH, 1999) identifies national guidance for recruitment and selection for Nurse Consultant posts, along with an outline of the key parameters and expectations of the role. The professional bodies, such as the College of Occupational Therapists (2003), have issued guidelines for managers and aspiring therapists to help to explain the professional expectations and responsibilities. In spite of this, the duties covered by NTC roles remain varied as local interpretation and local bids have often led to specific responsibilities being identified.

In some areas, NTC posts may be influenced by the extent of implementation of extended or specialist practice. The move from Specialist to Consultant has been discussed; Jones (2002) suggests that five years in specialist practice should be required before individuals are considered for Consultant roles, whereas others have stated the requirement as eight years (NHSE, 2001). Specialist practitioners have responsibility for a specific caseload and expertise in that area; part of their preparation for the NTC role will help them to develop the other skills that will be required for the post. These may include postgraduate study, continued professional development and support from managers.

Policy implementation, lack of systematic planning or resourcing

The national agreements for these posts did not bring with them new funding so posts have had to be funded from existing local resources, for example from redesigning or reconfiguring new services (Chartered Society of Physiotherapy, 2002). Posts have been established to tackle national initiatives as well as locally to address specific needs. This lack of national planning may go some way towards explaining the slow development of these posts as each has had to be bid for and negotiated individually. This may also explain the rather uneven pattern of development across the country in terms of both posts and focus.

Organisational factors, developing a supportive workplace

The key to the success of new roles is the context of their development; Wilson-Barnett (2003) believes that the support and vision of managers is required if posts are to be successful. Opposition may result from professional rivalry or threat, and new NTCs could be seen to be vulnerable as it will be largely up to them to determine the post's parameters. The interpretation of the four key principles of the post will be, by the very nature of their design, diverse and complex, resulting in very different posts. Specialist posts vary widely in structure, process and outcomes, and NTCs will echo this as they continue to develop in practice (Zwanziger et al, 1996; Dawson and Benson, 1997; Daly and Carnwell, 2003).

Activity 1.2 *Feedback*

Identifying the differences between Nurse/Therapist Specialists and NTCs

There are similarities and differences between Specialist and Consultant posts. These should be viewed not in terms of what one does differently, better, more or less than the other, but in the way in which each significantly and essentially contributes to improving patient care. The impact on the wider outcomes of a service's efficiency and effectiveness is also important.

CONCLUSION

The introduction of the NTC post as part of the modernisation reforms is exciting and timely for the health professions. The four key roles – expert practice, leadership, education and research – are important as services are redesigned and new ways of working are introduced across the health sector. NTCs will require the support of local teams, management and government in implementing this role in order to fulfil the expectations that we have all looked forward to for many years.

SUMMARY OF KEY POINTS

- A combination of societal, political and professional factors has contributed to the introduction of the NTC post.
- The NTC will be part of the reorganisation and reconfiguration of services as one aspect of the modernisation agenda.
- The success of the NTC depends on the creation of good, shared working relationships within teams.
- The NTC will be able to challenge current practice and be involved in new ways of delivering services.
- There are similarities and differences between Specialist and Consultant roles. They should be viewed both separately and together as both contribute to the quality of patient care and service delivery.
- The individual will have practical issues to resolve within the workplace.

RECOMMENDED READING

McSherry R, Bassett C (2002) *Practice Development in the Clinical Setting: A Guide to Implementation*. Nelson Thornes Ltd, Cheltenham.

Manley K (2001) *Consultant Nurse: Refining the Concept, Clarifying Process and Outcomes*. Royal College of Nursing, London.

REFERENCES

Adams A, Pelletier D, Nagy S et al (1997) Determining and discerning expert practice: a review of the literature. *Clinical Nurse Specialist* 11(5):217–222.

Benner P (1984) *From Novice to Expert: Excellence and Power in Clinical Nursing Practice.* Addison-Wesley, Menlo Park, California.

British Dietetic Association (2002) *Dietetic Consultant Posts Your Questions Answered.* www.bda.uk.com/

Browne DG (1996) Understanding barriers to basing nursing practice upon research: a communication model approach. *Journal of Advanced Nursing* 21:154–157.

Chartered Society of Physiotherapy (2002) *Physiotherapy Consultant (NHS): Role, Attributes and Guidance for Establishing Posts, PA56.* CSP, London.

College of Occupational Therapists (2003) *COT/BAOT Briefings – Occupational Therapy Clinical Specialist.* COT, London.

Creasia LJ, Parker B (1996) *Conceptual Foundations of Professional Nursing Practice.* Mosby, London.

Daly W, Carnwell R (2003) Nursing roles and levels of practice: a framework for differentiating between elementary, specialist and advancing nursing practice. *Journal of Clinical Nursing* 12(2):158–167.

Dawson J, Benson S (1997) Clinical nurse consultants: defining the role. *Clinical Nurse Specialists* 11(6):250–254.

Department of Health (1992) *The Patient's Charter; Raising the Standards.* Stationery Office, London.

Department of Health (1993) *The Citizens Charter.* Stationery Office, London.

Department of Health (1997) *The New NHS – Modern, Dependable: Executive Summary.* HMSO, London.

Department of Health (1999a) *Nurse, Midwife and Health Visitor Consultants: Establishing Posts and Making Appointments.* Health Service Circular HSC 1999/217. HMSO, London.

Department of Health (1999b) *Making a Difference: Strengthening the Nursing, Midwifery and Health Visiting Contribution to Health and Healthcare.* HMSO, London.

Department of Health (2000) *The NHS Plan: A Plan for Investment, a Plan for Reform.* HMSO, London.

Department of Health (2002) *Delivering the NHS Plan: Next Steps on Investment, Next Steps on Reform.* HMSO, London.

Department of Health (2003a) *Agenda for Change – proposed agreement.* HMSO, London.

Department of Health (2003b) *Health Sector Workforce Market Assessment.* Skills for Health, London.

Dineen M, Walshe K (1999) Incident reporting in the NHS. II. *Health Care Risk Report* 5(7):17–19.

Dowling S, Martin R, Skidmore P, Doyal L, Cammeron A, Lloyd S (1996) Nurses taking on junior doctors work: a confusion of accountability. *British Medical Journal* 312 (7040):1211–1214.

Greenough CG, Murray MM, Holmes M (1997) *Golden Helix Innovation in Health Care.* South Tees Acute Trust Submission, Golden Helix Organisation, Middlesbrough GHA/97/522.

Hargadon J (2001) Changing Workforce programme. *HR Directors Bulletin,* Feb:1–5, London.

Jones P (2002) Consultant nurses and their potential impact upon health care delivery. *Professional Nurse* 1(2):39–40.

Kelly LY, Joet LA (1995) *Dimensions of Professional Nursing*, 7th edn. McGraw Hill, London.

McSherry R, Bassett C (2002) *Practice Development in the Clinical Setting: A Guide to Implementation*. Nelson Thornes Ltd, Cheltenham.

McSherry R, Haddock J (1999) Evidence based health care: its place within clinical governance. *British Journal of Nursing* 8(2):113–117.

Manley K (2001) *Consultant Nurses: refining the concept, clarifying process and outcomes*. Royal College of Nursing Institute, London.

Meeting the Challenge 2000. http://www.doh.gov.uk/meetingthechallenge/index.htm/

Morris M, Herriot S (1994) RCN report highlights the limitations of the Patient's Charter. *British Journal of Nursing* 3(9):440–441.

National Health Service Executive, Trent Cancer Nurses Allied Health Professionals Advisory Group (2001) *Nurse Specialists, Nurse Consultants, Nurse Leads: The Development and Implementation of New Roles to Improve Cancer and Palliative Care. An Advisory Report*. NHS Executive, London.

NHS National Nursing Leadership Programme (2003) Nurse Consultants, National Nursing Leadership Project, www.modern.nhs.uk/

Nurse Practitioner United Kingdom (1999) *What is a Nurse Practitioner: Your Questions Answered*.

Pilling A (2003) A nurse led service for acute exacerbation of COPD. *Nursing Times* 99(26):32–34.

Richley W (2000) The rise of the specialist nurse. *Nursing Management* 7(8):36–37.

Royal College of Nursing (1994) *Uncharted Territory: Public Awareness of the Patient's Charter*. Royal College of Nursing, London.

Shuttleworth A (1992) Will the Charter work? Readers' views on the Patient's Charter. *Professional Nurse* April:439–431.

Sidani S, Irvine D (1999) A conceptual framework for evaluating the nurse practitioner role in acute setting. *Journal of Advanced Nursing* 30(1):58–66.

Smith R (1998) All changed, changed utterly: British medicine will be transformed by the Bristol case. *British Medical Journal* 316:1917–1918.

Sneed NV (1991) Power: its use and potential for misuse by nurse consultants. *Clinical Nurse Specialist* 5(1), Spring, 58–62.

UCLH NHS Trust (2003) *First UK MS Nurse Consultant developing high quality healthcare services for people with multiple sclerosis at UCLH*, www.uclh.org/ (accessed January 2004).

Wilkinson G, Miers M (1999) *Power and Nursing Practice*. Macmillan, London.

Wilson J (1996) Multi-disciplinary pathways of care series: a tool for minimising risks. *Health Care Risk Report* March:10–12.

Wilson J, Tingle J (1999) *Clinical Risk Modifications: A Route to Clinical Governance*. Butterworth Heinemann, Oxford.

Wilson-Barnett J (2003) *A Preliminary Evaluation of the Establishment of Nurse, Midwife and Health Visitors Consultants*. Florence Nightingale School of Nursing and Midwifery, Kings College, London.

Zwanziger JP, Peterson MR, Finley LJ, Degroot SL, Busman LC (1996) Expanding the CNS role in the community. *Clinical Nurse Specialist* 10(4):1999–1202.

2 THE NURSE/THERAPIST CONSULTANT: SETTING THE PARAMETERS

Wendy Francis, Liz Holey and Rob McSherry

INTRODUCTION

This chapter focuses on the scope and parameters of the Nurse/Therapist Consultant (NTC) role and the potential impact it may have on the British National Health Service (NHS). It is intended that key issues such as power, empowerment, collaboration, authority, professional accountability and medico-legal concerns will be addressed through critical debate within the context of the government's NHS modernisation agenda.

SETTING THE PARAMETERS OF THE NTC

The emerging literature associated with the NTC role seems to indicate that the NTC's longevity depends on the clear identification of parameters that will determine the necessary personal and professional attributes of the post. It will be necessary for these to be clearly understood so that the NTCs can fulfil the expectations of the post both for themselves and for their employers and clients.

Activity 2.1   *Reflective question*

Setting the parameters of the NTC

Write down what you feel are the key issues in the development of personal and professional parameters for the NTC.

Read on and compare your findings with those in the Activity Feedback on page 30.

Parameters determine a point or a line, and in this case it is the personal and professional parameters determining the role of the NTC that are of concern (Figure 2.1).

Organisational conditions impacting on the NTC role in daily practice

The parameter referred to as 'professional' is centred primarily on ensuring that the individual NTC post is positioned within the wider aspects of the professional disciplines working within the organisation. This is essential in order to ensure clear working boundaries, demonstrating where accountability starts and stops. This in turn helps to clarify how much autonomy the individual has to act and work independently within the post.

'Personal' parameters are associated with ensuring that the individual NTC has the essential qualities and qualifications to carry out the roles and responsibilities of the post.

It is also important to note here that these parameters may interact, as differing internal and external conditions promote or hinder the efficiency and effectiveness of the NTC in post.

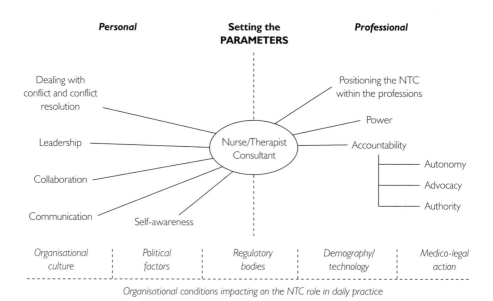

Figure 2.1 The importance of setting the parameters

SETTING THE PARAMETERS WITHIN THE PROFESSIONAL CONTEXT

Positioning the NTC within the professions

The Consultant role is well embedded in many other professions and generally relates to short-term, independent employment in an advisory capacity. This typically involves a professional being involved in, for example, advising another provider on setting up a service.

The medical profession has followed a unique system in which the term 'Consultant' has referred to a specific post that includes specialist clinical practice, team leadership, teaching and research. It carries a considerable degree of status and financial reward, and it is this model which the government has followed in its establishment of Consultant Practitioner posts (originally termed Nurse or Therapist Consultants). NTC posts mirror, to a large extent, the medical model of the consultant role, although it is unlikely in the foreseeable future that a health care professional other than a qualified doctor will have the *final* responsibility for a medical client group. These posts are, at the time of writing, still relatively new and carry with them the extra challenge of ground-breaking activity. There is the extra pressure on the post-holder in knowing that continued development and public and professional confidence will depend upon their early success.

The creation of the NTC posts can be seen within the context of a gradual shift away from a medically dominated power imbalance within the NHS. This has gradually been occurring since the introduction of the concept of general management and NHS Trusts with their Management Boards (DHSS, 1983). This was strengthened through the broader influences of health policy and government targets, economics and access and equity issues that have informed strategic managerial decisions. Clinical power is to a large extent the last bastion of medical dominance. Some of the advantages of extending Consultant roles beyond medicine include the redistribution of clinical power and influence, and having a wider range of professional perspectives informing clinical service decision-making. The shift of clinical responsibility towards other professionals has also been driven by the pressure arising from a reduction in junior doctors' hours.

It can be anticipated that introducing an NTC with a higher level of clinical leadership across a wider professional base may hasten NHS cultural change in areas such as evidence-based practice and interprofessional working. The impact of these new clinical leaders' experience may be that they will work very closely with patients and carers. Therapists, for example, who may work with a patient for long treatment sessions over an extended period of time, may be well placed to act as advocates for service users and carers. The true test and measure of the impact of the NTC role lies in seeing whether, within the parameters of the roles and responsibilities, they receive the power to control their destiny free of the influence and control of others.

Power: its relevance to the NTC

Power can be defined as 'the ability to do or act' (Collins English Dictionary, 1987). This sharing of clinical power, should, by definition, empower those who are new to it. To empower is defined by the Collins English Dictionary (1987) as 'to authorise or enable' and therefore involves the empowering of an individual or group, which then becomes 'empowered'. The term 'empowering' holds positive connotations such as releasing or sharing roles and responsibilities, whereas 'power' can be seen to be a negative way of viewing hierarchical authority, which can be used to restrict the freedom of others.

Although professionals often glibly refer to their empowerment of clients, 'empowerment' suggests that the process involves a passive recipient, which undermines the concept. It may be more accurate to describe professionals as enabling individuals to *become* empowered as empowerment is surely an active process that individuals or a group must achieve for themselves. Empowerment can be externally facilitated, but only the individual can be responsible for personal empowerment (Ridgeway and Wallace, 1994). These new roles therefore simply offer a structural mechanism via which professional groups may become empowered – if they choose to grasp the opportunity and use it to full effect.

It will, however, be very disempowering to clients/patients and their carers if attention becomes drawn to the professionals themselves. The NHS modernisation agenda aims to push power into communities through a development of primary care and a reconfiguring of funding flows whereby primary care providers become the purchasers, from acute NHS Trusts, of services they cannot provide for themselves.

User involvement in service design and delivery is a central ideal and should ensure that the needs of patients become more important than those of professionals. This has not, however, always been the case. NTCs need to concentrate their efforts on using their role to empower service users rather than focusing on empowering their professions. The challenges and difficulties facing NTCs lie in seeing whether the art of empowering others can be mastered through realising the potential of their role and responsibilities within the remit of their own professional accountability.

Realising the NTC post through professional accountability

The importance of exploring and reviewing professional accountability is an essential requirement in ensuring the efficiency and effectiveness of the NTC post. The principles associated with accountability argued by Glover (1999) are integral to and emergent within the NTC position. This is because of the post's strong association with and affiliation to practice. For example, within this context, the boundaries surrounding accountability seem to be based on three key factors (Glover, 1999):

- patients expect that, by virtue of the NTCs' training and position, they will be answerable to the patient while he or she is in their care
- accountability arises from training and education, which explains why the notion is present in some jobs and not others, knowledge being essential to justify why an event took place
- accountability and authority are interdependent, a greater degree of accountability being expected of those with greater authority, such as NTCs.

The need to be professionally accountable creates an imperative for NTCs to practise competently within their code or rules of professional conduct and to meet the standards of practice. According to Dimond (1995), accountability extends beyond professional practice. In exercising a duty of care, the practitioner is ultimately accountable to the public through criminal law, to the employer through contract law, contract of employment and job description, and to the patient through a duty of care and common and civil law. This is of interest because of the current awareness of the need to protect the public. This follows the findings of recent enquiries into unethical and even criminal practice within the boundaries of the NHS. Copp (1988) challenges the idealism associated with the contract of employment and the exercising of professional accountability by suggesting that, for NTCs to be accountable, they must have autonomy of action and authority to act within their defined role. This is a particular issue when the fear of litigation and reprisal in today's high-volume, low-cost health care service reduces an NTC's confidence to exercise autonomy and authority.

Taking the above parameters of professional accountability within the scope and remit of the NTC post, accountability seems to be associated with three important aspects: autonomy, advocacy and authority.

Autonomy within the NTC role

A high level of professional autonomy is needed for those undertaking these roles. This is currently variable across the different professions, as indicated by the Department of Health's 10 key roles for allied health professionals (AHPs) (DoH, 2003b) and 10 key roles for nurses (DoH, 1999a). The roles of the AHP include being a first point of contact, diagnosing, requesting and assessing diagnostic tests and drug prescribing, and playing an active role in strategic planning. Nurses' roles include referring for diagnostic tests, running clinics and admitting and discharging patients from hospital. Dieticians and speech and language therapists have had degree-level entry qualifications and independent practice for a number of decades. Other AHPs, for example physiotherapists and occupational therapists, have long been able to be involved in a patient's diagnosis and treatment without the need for referral to or review by a medical practitioner. This is normal practice for self-employed private practitioners, for example. Others, such as radiographers, are enjoying a more recent but rapid increase in the extension of their professional responsibilities, including reporting on medical images.

For nursing, professional autonomy has been growing more gradually, presumably partly because of different emphases and levels of preregistration education programmes. It is also partly due to the fact that the NHS is a biomedically based organisation and that the distinctive and primary role of the nurse is in providing care rather than diagnosis and treatment. The evidence offered by Buckenham and McGrath (1983), Orlando (1987) and Jennings (1986) shows that, throughout history, nursing has struggled to become 'independent', both in making decisions and in instigating or controlling practices central to patient care, because of the influences of other professional groups such as medicine, administration and management. If the latter situation continues to prevail within existing NHS cultures and professional disciplines, the notion of the NTC having autonomy to work independently may prove difficult and challenging in some areas of the NHS.

So what are the characteristics of an autonomous or independent professional? Corwin (1965) has characterised independent professional status in terms of six key attributes (Box 2.1).

Box 2.1   Characteristics of independent status (adapted from Strauss, 1963)

- Extensive formal training
- A high degree of skill and expertise applied in a specialised way
- A low degree of standardisation, with the profession utilising various alternative procedures for successful performance
- Decision-making based on training and expertise
- Client-orientated practice, involving aiding and assisting the client
- A college orientation, with colleagues and professional associations possessing sanctioning power

---

Adopting Corwin's (1965) characteristics of what constitutes an independent professional is important if autonomy is to be achieved within the role and responsibilities of the NTC. The autonomy conferred through professional status as identified by Corwin (1965) is essential to the future survival of these posts. The role and responsibilities of the NTC within the context of a modernising NHS will thrive in a health care environment, which enables practitioners to display and action the key points identified by O'Grady (1986) (Box 2.2).

Box 2.2   Creating an environment conducive to promoting authority within the NTC post (adapted from O'Grady, 1986)

- The freedom to function independently
- A sense of support from peers and governing bodies
- Clear explanations of the work environment
- Appropriate resources to practise effectively
- An open organisational culture

As we discussed in Chapter 1, it is evident from the information provided by Corwin (1965) and O'Grady (1986) that, for professionals to be autonomous (having the power or right to self-govern, without interference from other professions or administrative forces), they need the freedom and authority to act independently (Kelly and Joet, 1995). Independence in this context refers to the ability to control practice.

The importance of control and empowerment
When considering the emerging NTC post, it is important to remember that the historical lack of control, with subsequent feelings of being disempowered and devalued, has helped to fuel a protectionism of professional roles and skills. One natural evolution away from rigid and competitive professional boundaries is the development of shared working relationships in which collaboration is effective and mature. For this to be truly effective, multidisciplinary teams will

make way for interprofessional teams in which skill-sharing across professional boundaries becomes normal accepted practice. This will benefit the patient in that a professional visiting a patient at home may carry out a mixture of interventions that have traditionally 'belonged' for example, to a nurse, a physiotherapist or an occupational therapist. Adequate training and rigorous clinical governance would make the original professional background of the practitioner irrelevant.

The success of this approach will depend on mutual respect for professional differences as well as on an internalised, growing confidence and security rooted within NTCs themselves rather than being derived from a professional identity. Working beyond and outside these roles will to an extent remove individuals from their professional security blanket. *Making a Difference* (DoH, 1999a) and *Meeting the Challenge* (DoH, 2000a), as well as the practitioner's 10 key roles, all give NTCs permission to grow in a variety of professional ways and to become empowered to act more autonomously than has been previously encouraged within the NHS. The true measure of autonomy for the NTC will no doubt be associated with how boundaries are, from the outset, set or marked out.

The need for boundary clarifications

The establishment of an autonomous *role* is even more radical within the framework of the NTC and difficult to achieve in today's NHS, where all roles share a degree of definition, boundaries being defined for reasons of safety and organisational control. This is appropriate in a situation in which both clinical risk and financial accountability are subject to necessarily tight control. The NTC role is one in which a high degree of autonomy exists within potentially flexible boundaries. It is, for example, possible to have autonomy in target-setting and in identifying the evidence against which the success of the post will be measured. Different personality types will respond in different ways to this, some individuals valuing the freedom, others finding it highly uncomfortable and stressful. Potential or existing NTCs best suited to this flexibility are those who seem to thrive on the elements identified in Box 2.3.

Although this aspect of the role is essential, some of the earlier Nurse Consultants reported experiencing problems in defining their role and setting out

---

Box 2.3   Elements attributed to suit the flexibility of the NTC post

- Self-motivation
- Self-management
- Working to high personal and professional standards
- Demonstrating that strategic targets have been met
- Dynamic, continuous professional development
- Self-reflection
- Independent working
- Demonstrating a high level of achievement

---

the boundaries for themselves and others. There was an element of feeling 'thrown in the deep end' and left to discover their role for themselves (Guest, 2001). This emphasises the need for a certain type of person (with some or all of the elements outlined in Box 2.3), who can be thrown into this situation and truly embrace the concept of autonomy. Trust and commitment from across the organisation are essential to ensure that opposing strategies are not initiated, either by managers or by other professionals elsewhere in the system (Morgan, 1998). It is essential that all activity is aimed towards organisational priorities and the meeting of targets so that decisions are not overruled or initiatives blocked.

Within the NTC role, a high level of autonomy brings with it a high level of accountability. In this instance, accountability depends on the NTC being familiar with where the boundaries start and stop. Is the post-holder, for example, sufficiently informed about the evidence to ensure that the best available care, treatment or intervention is being delivered and evaluated within the scope and remit of the post? Within the scope and range of accountability, it is imperative that NTCs are aware of the need to become professionally responsible. Being professionally responsible is important for ensuring the effectiveness of the care, treatment or interventions provided at the level of operation of the NTC either within or outside the organisation (Lo Biondo-Wood and Haber, 1990).

The establishment of boundaries and parameters is essential so that NTCs have the fitness and purpose to practise or work independently and collaboratively if required. It could be argued that initial fitness for *practice* is conferred through graduation from an educational programme that confers eligibility for registration with the Health Professions Council, the Nursing and Midwifery Council or the General Medical Council, as appropriate. The maintenance of fitness for *purpose* requires NTCs to maintain competence through the changing demands and changing responsibilities of their work via a process of continuous professional development. This competence may be externally judged if NTCs are held accountable for their actions through being answerable and responsible for the outcome of their professional conduct (Pennel, 1997).

New, developing roles in health and social care, such as that of the NTC, require post-holders to work beyond their traditional scope of practice. It is understandable that Strategic Health Authorities (SHAs) may be concerned to make sure that clinical governance is not compromised. Individuals will need constantly to update and extend their skills just to stay competent in an ever-changing environment of increasing complexity. In the NTC role, many skills, particularly the important communication and 'people' skills, will be developed experientially, so evidence that they have been developed is based on outcome rather than educational certification. It could be argued that risk assessment and risk management, rather than just the management of all extended scope of practice roles, should therefore be more integral and explicit in their practice. The latter again reinforces the need for clarifying roles and expectations about where the roles' boundaries and parameters of start and stop.

In brief, it is essential that NTCs develop their knowledge, skills, understanding of the importance of professional accountability in promoting autonomous practice, and understanding of how personal attributes and role/boundary clarification(s) can influence this. The next important aspect associated with professional accountability is that of advocacy.

Advocacy and the NTC

Any discussion of power within the context of the NTC is incomplete without some consideration of advocacy. Teasdale (1998) defines 'advocacy' as influencing those who have power on behalf of those who do not. It is about advancing both human and legal rights in a supporting and protective way and is required when people feel vulnerable and powerless. In health and social care, advocacy has an established role in the field of mental health and learning disabilities, and is used formally in the judicial system (Carter, 2002). Any professional who has spoken out for patient needs perhaps on an individual basis has acted as an advocate.

Advocacy is also undertaken when contributing to service development, by offering, for example, a service user perspective during discussions involving efficiency and cost-effectiveness. In traditional health and social care, the professional is in possession of power, and either the effectiveness of communication, the culture or the organisational structures may have a promoting or disempowering effect on the power balance. Modernisation aims to reverse this. It is intended that giving patients a voice and an involvement in decisions about the running of services will empower them through the redistribution of power. The effect of this will, however, be limited unless *respect* is also equal. The professional must respect the patients' views, opinions and experience, in equal measure to that afforded in the opposite direction. An imbalance here is likely to increase the greater the mismatch in terms of social class, wealth and culture. NTCs can be important here: they speak on behalf of groups of staff and service users, rather than individuals, and can have a significant impact when attempting to drive changes in service design, ensuring that the patients' perspective is encompassed in a genuine rather than tokenistic way.

NTCs can also act as advocate for the profession – not just by empowering professionals to have confidence in themselves, but also by demonstrating that they can work in new and more challenging ways, in short by showing that the demands of clinical governance can be met. The NTC should be a champion for the belief that where parameters exist only as a result of tradition, they are there to be blurred. The role of the NTC in this therefore lies in influencing, facilitating and then supporting the development of a good professional service.

Actioning the NTC post within the context of professional accountability: authority

Authority may be recognised as a component of the NTC status but, as we argue later with regard to the personal parameters of the post, leadership is an integral and integrated part of authority. Levels of authority will be strengthened by a respect for the role but even more so by an earned respect for the individual. Morgan (1998) succinctly states that the level of authority one has is dependent on one's colleagues. This would make a sizeable difference, especially as the NTC sits outside the established structure of line management so does not always have authority through line management responsibilities.

This fits with Mullins' (2002) definition of the functional relationship of authority, which applies to the relationship between people in specialist or advisory positions, and line managers and their subordinates. The NTC provides a common service across the organisation but has no direct authority over those using the service. This concept of authority describes clearly one of the key components of the NTC's role. It is essential that conflict between the function of the NTC and management expectation is avoided as the resulting dissonance created for staff would be destructive. Urwick (2002, in Mullins, 2002) states that there should be a clear line of authority to every individual and that creative ways must be found to impart authority. The NTC in some ways sits alongside, rather than within, these lines of authority, and although the role itself suggests authority as associated with senior roles, this has to be earned on an individual basis. It would be expected that those individuals meeting the criteria for these roles would already, from their apparent personal and professional standards, have exhibited the ability to take on authority.

Activity 2.2   Reflective question

How an NTC achieves autonomy and authority within an organisation

Write down how you think the NTC achieves autonomy and authority within an organisation.

Read on and compare your findings with those in the Activity Feedback at the end of this section.

Having completed Activity 2.2, you might wonder how some NTCs achieve autonomy and authority within an organisation given that they do not have direct line management responsibility. By reading and reviewing Box 2.4, we can see how this can be achieved. The NTC achieves authority through the utilisation of a diverse range of personal, interpersonal and clinical skills and experience in working towards achieving authority within the role.

Box 2.4   NTC skills used to demonstrate the achievement of authority within the scope and remit of the post

- Using situational leadership strategies
- Working closely with other staff to discuss patient needs
- Demonstrating expert practice
- Providing consultancy role for managers and their staff
- Including managers in the development of new initiatives, and involving them in relevant steering groups and partnership work

---

For those in the early (Nurse) Consultant posts, authority was partly earned through the need to justify the appointment and partly in order to help other nurses to understand what was different about the role from that of, for example, Extended Scope Nurse Practitioners. This helped to reduce the suspicion and threat arising from these new posts. Sadly, some real hostility was experienced from within the nursing profession, perhaps because of personal envy or a recognition of missed opportunities. The legitimacy of the role, as well as its authority, had to be worked at. These are, however, common, temporary aspects of coping with change and are perhaps as much an indictment of how change is managed in the NHS as of the nurses themselves. This brings the discussion back to the theme of empowerment – personal and professional empowerment will enable individuals to manage personal change more effectively (Ridgeway and Wallace, 1994), whereas disempowerment can feed into a reluctance to, or even a fear of, change.

In summarising this section on setting the parameters of the NTC within the context of the professional, three important dimensions are emerging that will influence the future direction of these posts:

- positioning the NTC within the professions
- power
- accountability.

Activity 2.2   Feedback

How an NTC achieves autonomy and authority within an organisation

It is evident, according to Box 2.4 above, that several strategies are employed by NTCs to achieve autonomy and authority within their organisation. These essentially relate to seeking the respect and permission of other colleagues and users to perform a role to the highest standard through effective leadership, taking into account the unique organisational culture and working environment.

Having identified the importance of setting the professional parameters of the NTC post, we will now focus on the personal parameters.

SETTING THE PARAMETERS WITHIN THE PERSONAL CONTEXT

According to Figure 2.1 above, five primary dimensions associated with the setting of personal parameters are emerging:

- dealing with conflict and conflict resolution
- leadership
- collaboration through partnerships
- communication
- self and self-awareness.

It is the intention of this section to focus specifically on the first three dimensions because the authors feel that communication and self-awareness are topics discussed in detail in other contemporary literature.

Dealing with conflict and conflict resolution

Dealing with conflict and conflict resolution is emerging as a key debate central to the establishment and operationalisation of the NTC post in daily practice. Conflicts seem to be originating in organisations where the cultures and working environment have not been prepared to receive the posts or indeed informed of the key necessities and remits of the posts. This failure to communicate and market the NTC posts does not help to ensure a smooth transition into the post. Tensions and frustrations are emerging between and within professional groups and disciplines because the parameters and scopes of the NTC posts have not been adequately set. The culmination of the failure to communicate and share information about the posts is that health and social care professionals begin to divide over power and control.

Power conflicts may continue to create frustrations for NHS staff as the principles inherent in the modernisation plans are rolled out into practice. For example, as new ways of working are introduced, skill-sharing will increase between different grades of staff – between registered professionals and health care assistants and assistant practitioners, as well as between AHPs and nurses taking on skills and responsibilities previously undertaken by the medical profession. This raises concerns about clinical governance and how patient outcomes are affected (Gibbs et al, 1991; Buchan and Ball, 1991). It also highlights political concerns of replacing more highly qualified and highly paid staff with a cheaper workforce (Bevan and Stock, 1991).

Some of these issues are being addressed through the promised provision of foundation degrees via the National Health Service University for assistant practitioners and others. Similarly, the new pay spine identified through the *Agenda for Change* (DoH, 2003a) is designed to offer a mechanism for a more appropriate rewarding of the actual job and responsibilities undertaken, rather than purely basing pay and conditions on qualifications, knowledge and experience. Although research has shown that higher nursing grades give a better quality of care (Jolley and Brykczynska, 1995), the insufficient capacity in the NHS at a time of growing demand will ensure that role redesign will continue within the NHS. It is certain that this change and its effect on traditional power structures will be uncomfortable for many. The NTC has a significant leadership role to play in facilitating some of this radical change and in influencing the culture, which has maintained traditional power structures at the expense of better patient services.

We have previously argued and demonstrated that advocacy does not come without risks. As advocacy is about power, there is considerable potential for conflict. The NTC will be called upon to consider professional, service and patient needs and will have to make fine judgements about the invisible lines between these interests. NTCs will need to balance professional wants with patient needs, which may be complementary but are perhaps more often in conflict. Professional group X, for example, may want to continue working in a particular way because this is the traditional method and may benefit their status and authority. However, sharing those skills with another professional may ensure that a much larger number of patients benefit from the same intervention. Both patients and professionals may think that they require advocacy, but, in the spirit of modernisation, it is clear that the NTC has a responsibility to be the patient's advocate and a professional's diplomat.

Constructive conflict management is an approach whereby managers (and this equally applies to NTCs), who are in a position to create conflict, can instead have a positive influence on conflict. For this, they must have authority, responsibility for needs and quality, a co-ordinating and facilitating role and accountability. Dealing with conflict in a constructive way is effective, active and creative (Crawley, 1992). This is a skill that can be learned, just like any other. It is necessary for the NTC to stand back, adopt a wide overview and exercise objective judgement.

The issues fuelling any conflict often run deeper than those which are immediately apparent. Defining them and assisting those involved to recognise them may be an essential first step in solving the conflict. The breadth of the NTCs' roles means that they are able to effect a more permanent contribution through strategies such as team-building (Kindler, 1988). The style of communication employed may make the difference between the NTC making an important diplomatic contribution, inadvertently worsening the situation or, possibly more likely, having no significant impact.

Covey (1989) recommends the win/win approach. Negotiating must start with an understanding of the opposite position – i.e. identifying the issues from everyone's perspective (empathetic listening). A solution should be suggested that offers all sides the opportunity to 'win' something out of the situation. This is more than just compromise: it involves a positive gain by everyone involved. A disagreement over physical space in an interprofessional team could be solved by a model of sharing that offers a previously absent benefit – a more comfortable sitting area or better access to administrative staff or storage space. Having the knowledge, skills and experience to resolve and indeed prevent conflicts of interest may help to ensure good interprofessional teamwork and the establishment of robust partnerships.

Collaboration through partnership

NHS advance circular 1999/217 (NHS Executive, 1999) states that, in order to deliver better services, the NTC role will be crucial in influencing other disciplines across *intra-* as well as *inter*-organisational boundaries. This cross-boundary and interagency working can be complex for some NTCs, for example in fields such as public health or children's services. In user-centred services, client care needs rarely fit neatly into organisational structures; instead, they often cross different clinical areas, divisions, agencies and voluntary and statutory organisations.

Developing and working within partnerships will provide the best approach to delivering effective continuous patient care in such situations.

Although formalised professional partnerships are expanding through initiatives such as Children Centres, Connexions, Sure Start and New Deal for Communities, some NHS organisations will require organisational development programmes to assist them in embracing the elements of effective partnerships.

The Working Partnership (Markwell et al, 2003) explains that good partnership working can:

- generate solutions to problems that single agencies cannot solve
- improve the services that local communities receive
- enhance the co-ordination of services across organisational boundaries
- avoid waste for duplication and gaps in services, thus making better use of existing resources.

Given that collaboration and partnership-working are difficult concepts for organisations to address, and that many of the outcomes will depend on the robustness of the partnership, the factors outlined in Figure 2.2 would seem to be key to success. These are ambitious, albeit essential, components that prove difficult for organisations to adhere to on an equal basis. It is even more challenging to ensure that all these factors are implemented across a number of external agencies.

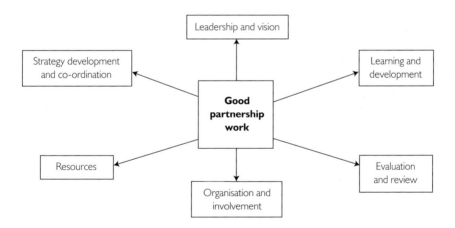

Figure 2.2 The importance of good partnership work (adapted from Markwell et al, 2003)

Parameters may present as boundaries, and the individual's personal and professional boundaries must be tackled first. This should be closely followed by tackling the organisation's internal boundaries, the internal boundaries of other organisations and the interagency boundaries. Where the aim is to develop effective partnerships upon which the success of cross-boundary working will depend, the challenge facing the NTC will take on an extra dimension.

Initiatives such as Sure Start and New Deal for Communities are bringing together new-style interprofessional teams involving wider configurations across the health and social services, and health and education. Staff may be seconded to work in such programmes. NTCs should provide support to ensure that while structures are becoming innovative, so is professional practice.

Collaboration can be defined as 'working in combination'. Collaboration, however, rarely happens naturally, and organisations internal and external to the NHS need to pay particular attention to promoting the concept of collaboration for it to be effective. It could be argued that personnel working within the NHS collaborate and work in partnership, but the reality is that while people perceive one profession to have authority over others, unequal partnerships will inevitably be generated. "The literature indicated that collaboration rarely happens either naturally, or as a result of exhortation and that attention must be paid to the process of promoting collaboration for it to be effective" (Taylor et al, 1998). Features essential for effective partnership-working are:

- effective communication through shared language
- trust
- commitment
- following a vision.

First, *shared language* is an issue because each profession i.e. medical/nursing and AHPs, has evolved its own jargon and set of abbreviations. Different professional groups sometimes use the same term to mean something different, which can create confusion. The potential for language problems is greater in multiagency communication, and as individuals may find this intimidating, valuable participation may be inhibited. The use of jargon is exclusive and can prevent the genuine and effective involvement of patients/clients, professionals and the public.

Second, *trust* is a central tenet of effective collaboration and has to be earned rather than assumed. The establishment of trust, which will ultimately determine the level and quality of the partnership work undertaken, must occur first in the development of any relationship. Conflict can often only be resolved if the team steps back from the problem and works on trust issues. Experience has shown that a useful approach lies in providing an emotionally safe environment, creating space to explore team dynamics and providing expertise in team development. Trust must be implicit when engaging with multidisciplinary teams. External mentoring and facilitation may be needed to achieve this; it may be that the NTC is not sufficiently 'outside' the team, requiring an external person to be involved to help with partnership work.

Third, *commitment* is needed for successful partnership-working. This commitment, however, has to be evident across all partners on an individual and organisational basis. It seems that organisations can unknowingly sabotage partnerships because of an organisational reluctance to change traditional policies and practices. This is often seen where an individual wishes to pursue an innovative approach to the development and delivery of a service. This may stretch the boundaries of current practice, and the parent organisation may be unwilling to let go of tradition. In such situations, the NTC's role is to provide expert knowledge, leadership and advocacy to influence and enable these new approaches. This can be highly stimulating as it means working with individuals and organisations to let go of power, a particular cross-agency issue. Agencies whose *raison d'être* has been to build strength and reputation from expertise and results must become prepared to share this expertise in an altruistic way. NTCs must provide the leadership to encourage non-traditional thinking and practice. It would be a mistake, however, to underestimate the vulnerability and loss that individuals may feel as a result of this process, a feeling that may also extend to patients participating in new approaches to health and health care delivery.

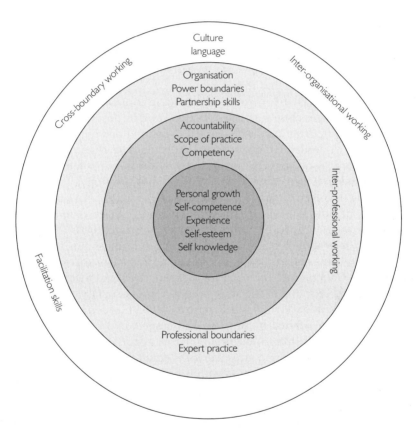

Figure 2.3   Achieving effective partnership within the NTC role

According to Figure 2.3, the NTC, in order to provide the leadership and vision element of effective partnerships, needs to possess a sound grounding in personal development, as illustrated by the inner circle of the diagram. To be confident in translating this to other agencies in the outer circle, the NTC also needs a fourth feature *a strong sense of the profession's vision* – the second circle – the organisation's vision being the third circle.

This figure illustrates that all four concepts of vision are needed, that the components are interrelated and that each circle influences and ripples out to the next. This concept can, in fact, be transferred to other areas of the NTC role. It is emerging that exploring the important role of collaboration and partnership is a way of judging the efficiency and effectiveness of the NTC role. Leadership will be integral to achieving change, and this is explored in the next section.

Leadership

It can be argued that the NTC role will be of limited effectiveness without a skilled leadership function and that this is the most challenging aspect of the role, challenging because it is the least easily defined, structured and evaluated part of the role. The acceptance that leadership is an integral component of clinical skill is new to the NHS. Despite a roll-out of Leading an Empowered Organisation training across the health care professions, anecdotal evidence suggests that the success with which individuals are developing leadership behaviours and transferring them into practice is variable.

But what is leadership? Current thinking in organisation science is that leadership is no longer closely attached to a position or post but is instead a set of behaviours resulting from personal characteristics and personal and professional development. Real leadership qualities are and should be observed at all levels of the organisation; associating leadership with position is no longer the current dogma. The NHS is becoming a decentralised organisation in which strategic power is being devolved from the Department of Health to SHAs and Foundation Trusts, financial power from Health Authorities to Primary Care Trusts (PCTs), and clinical power from doctors to other professionals. Although, in accountability terms, the NHS remains hierarchical, leadership is concerned with creating vision, being results driven, risk-taking and problem-solving. Writers such as Covey (1989) emphasise the need for self-reflection and awareness to ensure that personal success and leadership precedes professional leadership. Leider (1996) describes self-leadership as being the essence of leadership. His leaders are motivated by vision, ignited by purpose and empowered by values. It could be argued that leaders (directors and consultants) are concerned with 'doing the right thing', whereas managers are concerned with 'doing things right'.

The NTC needs the confidence – within defined parameters – with which to develop a vision that is aligned to the organisation's vision and the NHS Trust's clinical strategy. This should currently resonate with the government's modernisation vision. This is problematic where the NTC and the employing organisation are uncertain of the role and its objectives, reflecting a deficiency in the rigour with which the post was originally approved and in the leadership and visionary qualities of the individual NTC. It is also important that clinical objectives are not developed in isolation from the objectives of another clinical speciality as this has the potential to create conflict.

Cameron and Masterson (2000) have found that the development of new clinical roles has sometimes been influenced more by the availability of financial support rather than strategic direction. This has led to some early post-holders finding it hard to define the role, sometimes resulting in uncertainty and suspicion on the part of colleagues who were ill prepared to accept this new role.

Research by Guest (2001) identified that 51% of Nurse Consultant posts were filled from internal applications. This will be an advantage in terms of detailed organisational knowledge, enabling the NTC to establish relationships more quickly after taking up the post. It may, however, be more difficult to develop a new vision as this necessitates standing back, looking objectively at the issues and taking a strategic overview. The previous relationships and reputation enjoyed by the individual may be an asset, whereas any previous involvement in conflicts or unpopular decisions may be a disadvantage.

Where leadership skills are in evidence, the people surrounding the leader show a desire and willingness to be led, an effect that will be enhanced if the leader carries authority. Individuals have traditionally responded to the authority (which again demonstrates the overlap between the personal and professional parameters) conferred by the nature of the position. The new approaches, creating flatter organisational structures and relationships, mean that this can no longer be assumed. Mullins (2002) describes the different authority relationships that exist in organisations (Figure 2.4):

- line
- functional
- staff
- lateral.

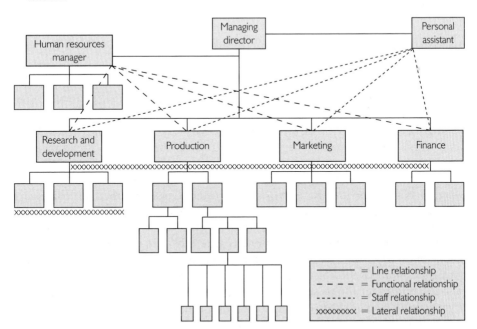

Figure 2.4 Illustrations of formal organisational relationships (*Management and Organisational Behaviour* 6th Edition, Laurie Mullins, Pearson Education Ltd © Laurie J Mullins 2002.)

When reviewing the role and remit of the NTC post and reflecting upon Figure 2.4, it seems that these are all important elements of overall accountability but come into play in different situations.

In summary, the personal aspects of setting the parameters of the NTC post are associated with the essential skills and attributes needed for the post. It is, however, imperative that the NTC explores these aspects of the role and responsibilites in order to avoid conflicts of power and interest. This will help to ensure the development of long, lasting and rewarding collaborations and partnerships. The latter is almost impossible without exploring one's own position and becoming self-aware within one's working culture and organisation. It is essential that appropriate personal and professional parameters are established. When measuring success, it is the impact of the individual that will be important.

The final section of this chapter briefly focuses on the conditions impacting on the NTC role in daily practice.

Activity 2.1 Feedback

Setting the parameters of the NTC

Setting parameters associated with the professional and personal dimensions of the NTC's role and responsibility is essential in order to delineate the scope and remit of the post(s) within the context of the organisation's culture and working environment.

CONDITIONS IMPACTING ON THE NTC ROLE IN DAILY PRACTICE

The conditions affecting the role of the NTC in daily practice have been outlined in some detail in Chapter 1 and are reiterated here. In Figure 2.1 above, five conditions – as opposed to barriers – have the potential to influence the NTC role in practice: organisational culture, political factors, regulatory bodies, demography/technology and medico-legal action. The authors have chosen the term 'conditions' as opposed to 'barriers' because of the negative connotations of the latter and its inappropriateness when referring to the NTC. 'Conditions' implies both good and not-so-good rather than carrying any negative or emotive weight. NTCs are highly important as change agents, both in enhancing confidence in the abilities of outside professionals and in facilitating cultural change from within the professional groups.

In order to promote advances in practice, the NTC will need to be aware of the importance of these conditions and the potential to promote or hinder the implementation of the role. Most of the conditions were highlighted in Chapter 1 so the remainder of this section will focus on expanding the condition 'medico-legal action', which has not yet been mentioned in much contemporary literature associated with the NTC.

Establishing the medico-legal parameters of the NTC

It has become clear that NTC posts are new and progressive, and fall outside traditional lines of authority, management and the acknowledged scope of daily professional practice. They inevitably involve a degree of creativity and therefore risk. So how safe are they in terms of the law? The professional is required to work within legal, ethical and moral frameworks in order that the public is protected. In the current situation of modernising health care, the old, prescribed ways of carrying out professional duties are becoming obsolete as professionals enjoy new levels of autonomy and are actually required to advance their practice and work in new ways within new teams and services. This situation is managed in the NHS through risk assessment and clinical governance, but how does the NTC ensure that new practice falls within the law?

Key to answering this question are the two concepts of competence and negligence. The NTC will face legal proceedings if a complaint is brought and upheld; in order to help counteract this, there should be protection from vexatious complaints through the screening procedure. It is generally assumed that genuine complaints will be avoided while the NTC remains competent, and competence must constantly be demonstrated through continuous professional development and training. The NTC will only be under real threat of prosecution or removal from the professional register if proved to be incompetent or negligent. Negligence is fairly clear and can be avoided if practice meets the minimum professional standards at all times. Developing practice may mean that the practitioner develops skills before the practice becomes enshrined in the written standards of the relevant profession. The courts work to the principle of the Bolam test, in which the standard expected of the 'ordinary skilled man' professing to have that skill will be established on the advice of expert witnesses (Dimond, 1999).

Proving competence is, however, more problematic, particularly if the practitioner is pioneering new ways of working. These may stretch the definitions of the professional's scope of practice and go beyond the written contract of employment. It is generally accepted that the new parameters become those agreed and supported by the organisation. This may involve having a written plan detailing objectives, with evidence that identified training needs have been met. It will also be important that robust and appropriate supervision arrangements are set up and risk management strategies identified for both the professions and the public. This should enable the NTC to demonstrate safe and competent practice.

CONCLUSION

In this chapter, we have attempted to focus on the scope and parameters of the role of the NTC by exploring the professional and personal dimensions of the role and how these are aligned to power, empowerment, professional accountability and leadership.

It is hoped that this chapter has served to set the context for others in this book, which go on to address the more specific components of this exciting and challenging role. The discussion has constantly veered from the professional and theoretical to the personal qualities of NTCs. The professional qualities of the NTC will be central to success in this role. These strategic level functions of leadership, empowerment and the capacity to drive change will be key elements of the new partnership-working in the NHS.

SUMMARY OF KEY POINTS

- Organisations engaged in establishing an NTC post should pay particular attention to the strategic objectives and the authority associated with the role.
- The integration of a new NTC should be carefully managed.
- The success of the NTC role will depend on leadership skills granted through authority. Authority in this instance is based on wisdom, personal knowledge, reputation and expertise (Mullins, 2002).
- The NTC must be a facilitator, suited to those who see themselves in a creative, specialist or professional role.
- The NTC will play an important part in advocacy and conflict resolution.
- The NTC will be in a position of strategic influence and power.

CASE STUDY 2.1	THE IMPORTANCE OF SETTING PARAMETERS: THE REFLECTIONS OF AN INAUGURAL NURSE CONSULTANT IN PUBLIC HEALTH

Wendy Francis Nurse Consultant in Public Health, Middlesbrough NHS RGN, RM, RHV, MA, PCT

Introduction: Getting started – putting my initial thoughts, feelings and reflections into context

I want you to experience the learning and development of my role in the first 3 years of being a nurse consultant (NC). When I first came into post, I explained to people that I was indeed a fledgling NC. I needed to learn to fly, and when you watch how a bird learns to fly you will begin to be able to appreciate my journey into becoming an adult NC.

The most challenging concept I needed to understand was that this was a completely new role, and being one of the first 50 in the country, I needed to create the role. It was a scary time, and I had to draw on the skills and experiences I had acquired throughout my nursing career to enable me to take on this challenging and exciting role. Each day I faced a new venture, possibly one that had not been achieved by a nurse before. I had to be willing to move out of my comfortable boundaries and experience new ways of working. You may wonder why I wish to allude to this journey. Well, the theme of this chapter is parameters and challenging established practices. It may help you to know that I, as an NC, experienced periods of uncertainty and wondered whether I had made the right career choice. One of my expectations was that I would now be expected to know everything because I suddenly had the title 'Consultant'. What took me and others time to digest was that, as there had not been an NC in the NHS before, the role still had to be defined. In order to illustrate this, I have outlined one of the initial questions that I had to consider: 'How easy is it to work across organisations when, traditionally within the NHS, there are fairly rigid and defined organisational boundaries?'

Historically, nurses keep within their clinical boundaries and generally work within a given discipline or are assigned to a particular ward. So asking an NC, who is generally steeped in an NHS background, to work across disciplines and organisations was, I felt, a great challenge

I will discuss the following key cornerstones that I developed in my role as an NC in public health:

- the national agenda
- the local agenda
- collaborative/partnership-working
- developing an educational training package
- shaping service provision.

The national agenda

When working in a Consultant role, it is crucial that a rational and robust argument is evident when undertaking any new initiatives, especially if one is pushing out traditional parameters. Therefore, the inception and development of the breast screening pilot within Middlesbrough PCT area was based on national priorities, which were targets laid down by *Saving Lives. Our Healthier Nation* (DoH, 1999b). *The NHS Plan* (DoH, 2000b) stated that the national target was 70% uptake for breast screening and that the eligible age for the NHS breast screening programme was to increase from 50–64 to 50–70 years of age.

The local agenda

It is important to link the national agenda to the local PCT or NHS Trust Agenda to determine which targets organisations need to prioritise. Indeed, in the Middlesbrough PCT, there were a number of GP practices that had an uptake of fewer than 70% of women attending for breast screening. I therefore felt there was a rational reason to develop a new way of working, across professional and organisational boundaries, that would increase better service provision for patients. The overall aim was to increase uptake in the practices with figures below 70% and also to have a holistic approach to enabling women to make informed choices to attend for screening.

Collaboration and partnership-working

It takes creative leadership to be confident to work across professional and agency boundaries, but it also requires the Consultant to have the scope to be autonomous. To deliver effective services, especially in public health, it is important to embrace all the elements of partnership and to take into consideration all the individuals who can influence the service delivery of the target population. Breast screening is usually seen to be a responsibility of clinical staff, and therefore only these staff would possibly access relevant training courses. I wanted to think more widely and consider other staff, professionals and agencies that could, with a bit of imagination, have an impact on the breast screening services. The people and organisations listed in Table 2.1 were therefore involved in the initiative.

Table 2.1   Those involved in the initiative

Health professionals	Other disciplines
GPs	Receptionists
Breast screening services	Ethnic minority peer educators
Community psychiatric nurses	Community groups
Health visitors	Community development workers
Midwives	Health promotion staff
Community/learning disability nurses	Practice managers
School nurses	

The first step in working with these individuals was to ascertain their level of knowledge, their attitudes, perception of breast cancer and breast screening, as well as to listen to their frustrations and possible barriers.

Developing an education and training package

From these consultations, a programme of workshops, tailor-made for all those identified, was developed. Some were delivered in GP surgeries, community centres, psychiatric premises and training venues.

A portfolio of documentation was produced that included the background to the initiative, statistical epidemiological data on breast cancer and screening uptake, the health belief model, barriers to attending for health care and information on the breast screening service. Also included was a protocol developed for the staff to follow which provided a uniform structured approach that was implemented in the practices. This piece of work ensured that all the staff were delivering the same message to women, thus preventing any patient confusion. Guidance on how to conduct a consultation with eligible women, for example those between the ages of 50 and 70, was also produced.

Shaping service provision

So how does the Consultant convince other agencies and professionals who may not have a direct role in breast screening to become involved?

This is all about working differently, being proactive and identifying any possible links for other staff. For example, community psychiatric nurses would not have thought about being a part of promoting breast screening to their patients. However, my expert knowledge of mental health, psychological and practical barriers and the process of breast screening enabled me to tailor the training and education package to suit their client group. I suggested what role they could take with women with enduring mental illness who were eligible for breast screening. We then discussed a strategy to empower the nurses to feel confident and competent to raise the issue of breast screening. The idea was that this would therefore enable their client group, who traditionally found it difficult to attend, to make an informed choice. This led to the community psychiatric nurses being able to offer support to their clients to attend, as they had an understanding of the process of breast screening and therefore the importance of attending.

It was planned to implement this initiative for 4–6 weeks (prior to the women receiving an invitation to attend for breast screening). The breast screening service would be inviting women in Middlesbrough over a period of 12–14 weeks, so throughout this time all those who had been trained were actively promoting breast screening and enabling women to make informed choices. Given that not all women come into contact with health care professionals, it was important to use other media to get the message across. This led to the development of the following:

- a laminated display, designed and produced for each clinical area
- a flyer advertising the service for community venues
- a local press release detailing information on breast screening, which was placed in the local newspaper.

This new way of working has enabled women to be more informed about breast cancer and the screening programmes, and the uptake of breast screening has increased in Middlesbrough. Also a good model of collaborative and partnership-working has enhanced the promotion of breast screening.

Conclusion: lessons learnt so far

This case study demonstrates the four key elements of the consultant's role, including working strategically across traditional professional and agency boundaries, and links with the elements illustrated in Figure 2.3 above: being self-confident (the inner circle), having the knowledge of knowing my expert practice (second circle), interprofessional knowledge and service provision (third circle) and finally the outer circle – working strategically across other organisations.

My role has been to influence future services, and because of the intensive proactive work undertaken, many women have had the opportunity to make practical suggestions towards reshaping the breast screening service. As a result of their comments and my close working with different agencies, the breast screening service is moving its mobile unit in order to be closer to communities that find it difficult to access the service. This will inevitably contribute towards better service provision for women eligible for breast screening.

The initiative was based on national research and local evidence, which informed the approach necessary for developing this service. Using my nursing expertise, and my knowledge of breast cancer and breast screening, I developed partnership-working at a strategic level and was able to help to design a new service appropriate for the people of Middlesbrough.

RECOMMENDED READING

Cameron A, Masterson A (2000) Managing the unmanageable? Nurse executive directors and new role developments in nursing. *Journal of Advanced Nursing* 31(5):1080–1088.

Crawley J (1992) *Constructive Conflict Management. Managing To Make a Difference.* Nicholas Brealey, London.

Teasdale K (1998) *Advocacy in Health Care.* Blackwell Science, Oxford.

REFERENCES

Bevan S, Stock J (1991) *Choosing an Approach to Reprofiling and Skill Mix.* Brighton, Institute of Manpower Studies.

Buchan J, Ball J (1991) *Caring Costs.* Brighton, Institute of Manpower Studies.

Buckenham EJ, McGrath G (1983) *The Social Reality of Nursing.* Health Science Press, Bristol.

Cameron A, Masterson A (2000) Managing the unmanageable? Nurse executive directors and new role developments in nursing. *Journal of Advanced Nursing* 31(5):1080–1088.

Carter J (2002) *The Legal and Clinical Risk Implications of Practice Development.* In McSherry R and Bassett C (2002) *Practice Development in the Clinical Setting.* Nelson Thornes Ltd, Cheltenham.

Collins W (1987) *Collins Universal Dictionary.* Readers Union Ltd, Glasgow.

Copp G (1988) Professional accountability: the conflict. *Nursing Times* 84(3):42–44.

Corwin R (1965) *The Professional Employee: A Study of Conflict in Nursing Roles.* In Skipper J and Leonard R *Social Interaction and Patient Care.* JB Lippincott Company, Philadelphia.

Covey S (1989) *The 7 Habits of Highly Effective People.* Simon & Schuster, London.

Crawley J (1992) *Constructive Conflict Management. Managing To Make a Difference.* Nicholas Brealey, London.

Department of Health (1999a) *Making a Difference.* Stationery Office, London.

Department of Health (1999b) *Saving Lives. Our Healthier Nation.* Stationery Office, London.

Department of Health (2000a) *Meeting the Challenge.* HMSO, London.

Department of Health (2000b) *The NHS Plan.* Stationery Office, London.

Department of Health (2003a) *Agenda for Change – proposed agreement.* HMSO, London.

Department of Health and Social Security (1983) *NHS Management Enquiry* (Griffiths Report). DHSS, London.

Dimond B (1995) *Legal Aspects of Nursing*. Prentice Hall, London.

Dimond B (1999) *Legal Aspects of Physiotherapy*. Blackwell Science, Oxford.

Gibbs I, McCaughan D, Griffiths M (1991) Skill mix in nursing: a selective review of the literature. *Journal of Advanced Nursing* 16:242–249.

Glover D (1999) *Accountability*. Nursing Times Monograph. Emap Healthcare, London.

Guest D (2001) *A Preliminary Evaluation of the Establishment of Nurse, Midwife and Health Visitor Consultants*. King's College, London.

Jennings BM (1986) Nursing science: more promise than threat. *Journal of Advanced Nursing* 11:505–511.

Jolley M, Brykczynska G (1995) *Nursing Beyond Tradition and Conflict*. Mosby, London.

Kelly LY, Joet LA (1995) *Dimensions of Professional Nurisng*, 7th edn. McGraw Hill, London.

Kindler HA (1998*) Managing Disagreement Constructively*. Kogan Page, London.

Leider RJ (1996) The ultimate leadership task: self-leadership. In Hasslebein F, Goldsmith M, Beckhard R (eds) *Leader of the Future*. Drucker Foundation, Jossey Bass, CA.

Lo Biondo-Wood G, Haber J (1990) *Nursing Research: Methods, Critical Appraisal and Utilisation*. Mosby, Toronto.

Markwell S, Watson J, Speller V, Platt S, Young T (2003) *The Working Partnership*. NHS Health Development Agency, London.

Morgan G (1998*) Images of Organisations*. Berrett-Koehler/Sage, San Francisco, USA.

Mullins LJ (2002) *Management and Organisational Behaviour*, 6th edn. Pearson Education Ltd.

National Health Service Executive (1999) *Nurse, Midwives, and Health Visitor Consultants – Establishing Posts and Making Appointments*. Health Service Circular 1999/217. NHS Executive, London.

Porter-O'Grady T (1996) cited in Creasia LJ, Parker B *Conceptual Foundations of Professional Nursing Practice*. Mosby, London.

Orlando JI (1987) Nursing in the 21st century: alternative paths. *Journal of Advanced Nursing* 12:405–412.

Pennel C (1997) Nursing and the law: clinical responsibility. *Professional Nurse* 13(3):162–164.

Ridgeway C and Wallace B (1994) *Empowering Change: the role of people management*. Institute of Personnel & Development, London.

Taylor P, Peckman S, Turton P (1998) *A Public Health Model of Primary Care – from Concept to Reality*. Public Health Alliance, Birmingham.

Teasdale K (1998) *Advocacy in Health Care*. Blackwell Science, Oxford.

3 Outlining the essential attributes of a nurse/therapist consultant: a role analysis

John Campbell and Sue Gavaghan

Introduction

The purpose of this chapter is to outline the essential attributes of a Nurse/Therapist Consultant (NTC) through a reflective role analysis. The differences between 'specialist' practitioners and NTC practice will be examined.

The NTC in the early years: a brief historical overview

In the early years of the NTC, there was an enormous diversity of focus, not only between specialist appointments, but also between individual appointments to posts with similar titles. The political drive to set these posts up created an impetus for the development of the roles within a basic framework, this basis framework being outlined in Box 3.1.

Box 3.1   The initial key delivery areas of the NTC post

The initial key delivery areas of the NTC post were associated with having advanced levels of:
- clinical practice
- professional leadership
- consultancy
- education training and development
- practice and service development
- research and evaluation
- delivering the clinical governance/modernisation agenda.

The emergent delivery areas highlighted in Box 3.1 demonstrate the key aspects of the NTC post, which are reinforced in several papers (e.g. Manley, 1997; Byrne, 2002). The limitation of this initial work led to a lack of enough detail to produce a comprehensive job specification.

The first requirement for applicants to these posts was that they should have sufficient vision and drive to be able to identify the opportunities and potential for the role within the organisation so it would not be seen as a 'Micky Mouse' post (Byrne, 2002). These pioneers have built on the initial foundations to produce a diversity of roles that are specific to locality requirements and needs. The posts that have had the most transparent function are those which have been aligned to the political objectives arising from the modernisation agenda. It is intended that the NTC should lead by example so junior staff have something to aspire to – the NTC should lead the way (Limb, 2003). The broad diversity of NTC posts that have been developed from the initial tranche of nursing appointments through to the most recent Therapist roles have at their heart the four key delivery areas:

- expert clinical practice
- leadership
- education
- research.

Of these four key delivery areas, expert clinical practice is central to the role of the NTC. Through a consolidation of practice with study to Master's or Doctorate level will come clinical credibility and expert clinical practice that will be firmly anchored within evidence-based practice. The NTC will be an individual who will be able to take on the challenges of the modernisation agenda with positive and strategic vision.

If the NTC is to be accepted, a positive role model is part of the key to success. This initially proved difficult as the political agenda met the shop floor, leading to some adverse publicity that focused on the high salaries offered by these posts rather than the opportunities for the growth of the profession. This led to the inappropriate label of 'Supernurse' from some of the nursing press (O'Dowd, 2000). Thus anyone who was prepared to take on this 'poisoned chalice' had not only to adapt to the strange new world of the NTC, but also to be aware of the cynicism, envy or fear that they might face from work colleagues, old and new, as articulated in Box 3.2.

Box 3.2   The anonymous colleague view point of the new role of the NTC

'I know this sounds ironic but it was a relief to find an ambivalent attitude to the post of Nurse Consultant. The people who admitted they did not know much about the posts, or who thought that it could be an idea that should be explored, offered at least some hope during the *"death-by-lunch"* interview session. The only alternative was reflected in the statement: "I'd rather spend the money that is being wasted on this, on some new equipment."'

Making a Difference (DoH, 1999a) and *Meeting the Challenge* (DoH, 2000a) identified the objectives of developing NTC roles as offering an opportunity to maintain clinical skills in clinical practice and offering an alternative career progression to staff with a strong clinical preference. Prior to this, the only opportunities were to follow a career pathway into education or management.

The focus on expert clinical practice as a central function of the NTC was strengthened in a Department of Health White Paper (1999b) stating that the posts in nursing and midwifery were required to involve working directly with patients, clients or communities for at least 50% of the time. How this was to be exercised and the weak definition of clinical caseload offered in the job specifications was sometimes unhelpful. Job descriptions have had a tendency to list competencies under the subheading of expert clinical practice but often confuse what are practice competencies and what are leadership or educational competencies.

The concept of nurses taking on a caseload remains in its infancy, although this has been a recognised part of a Therapist's role for some time. Job specifications may therefore remain premature unless there is clear remit that has been identified for NTCs. This remit must be accepted by the institutions prior to the appointments if a senior clinical career structure is to be achieved. The consequence may be an alternative definition of expert clinical practice for some allied health professionals (AHPs) and Nurse Consultants. The lack of direction in the job specifications regarding caseload management and expert clinical practice has led to the prescribed level of 50% of clinical time becoming ever more flexible and often involving patients only indirectly. This supports the argument that expert clinical practice can be better exercised within the remit of strategic leadership or education, as by practising at this macro level, there is an impact on a greater patient caseload.

This, however, shifts the emphasis of the NTC role to a leadership or strategic position, which puts the direct patient care focus at risk and may dissuade clinical practitioners from pursuing this career opportunity. Ultimately, the objectives set out in *Making a Difference* and *Meeting the Challenge* could be undermined. NTC applicants must be prepared to accept the caseload or expert clinical practice function from the outset of the application process with all of the agencies that have been involved in producing the job descriptions and specifications.

The differences between the Nurse/Therapist Specialist and the NTC were outlined in Chapter 1. Here we are looking at the NTC and will identify how these differences have been realised. A number of job descriptions and personal specifications from across the United Kingdom have been reviewed, and it appears that although expert clinical practice is key to all, the remaining three supporting areas should also be considered fundamental to the position of the NTC.

There are clear interrelationships between the delivery areas that will lead to a coherent whole (DoH, 1999b). The NTC must maintain the capacity for the delivery of each function to be weighted according to service and locality demands. With greater experience of what the NTC role has to offer, and what opportunities there are for role development, post-holders will need the potential to evolve with these changes. As service requirements develop, NTCs must continue to demonstrate that all four key functions are still integrated into their role.

Activity 3.1 *Reflective question*

Identifying the key roles of the NTC

Write down what you think the key roles of the NTC are.

Read on and compare your findings with those in the Activity Feedback at the end of this section.

The emerging key roles of the NTC that you have indicated in Activity 3.1 were highlighted in *Nurse, Midwife and Health Visitor Consultants: Establishing Posts and Making Appointments* (DoH, 1999b) and the Advance Letter (AL) Professions Allied to Medicine (PAM) (PTA) 2/2001 (DoH, 2001). The specific details and anticipated expectations of the NTC are clearly articulated in these documents.

In brief, it is evident that the NTC role was initially developed by the nursing profession but has now widened to include AHPs. The initial government documents provided some initial information identifying the key roles and responsibilities of these posts. The next section builds on this by comparing, through a role analysis, the key attributes identified in a range of NTC job descriptions with examples taken from a range of actual job descriptions advertised in the press over the period 2002–03.

Activity 3.1   Feedback

Identifying the key roles of the NTC

The four key roles of the NTC are:

- expert clinical practice
- professional leadership and consultancy
- research and evaluation
- education, training and development.

IDENTIFYING AND DESCRIBING THE ESSENTIAL ATTRIBUTES OF THE NTC

This section provides a role analysis of the NTC and the key attributes of the post.

Activity 3.2   Reflective question

The essential attributes of the NTC

Take some time to write down what you think the essential attributes of an NTC are.

Read on and compare your findings with those in the Activity Feedback at the end of this section.

From Activity 3.2, you will no doubt have established that the essential attributes associated with the NTC role can be classified into professional, interprofessional and personal. The remainder of this section focuses on explaining these key attributes.

Describing the professional attributes of the NTC

The emerging professional attributes of the NTC role appear to be centred on four key components identified in Figure 3.1.

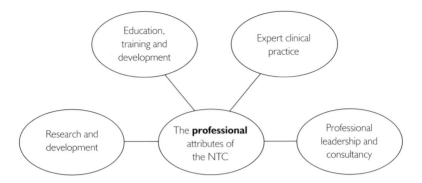

Figure 3.1   The professional attributes of the NTC

Expert clinical practice

All NTCs will be experienced senior clinicians who can demonstrate advanced knowledge and skills within a specific specialised or general field of practice. They will be responsible for complex caseloads, which may include undertaking technical or other clinical interventions that have traditionally been the remit of medical or other staff. These will not, however, be expected to be a principal element of the role, although the provision of expert advice may well be a key element, along with the development of protocols or standards.

The NTC will demonstrate a whole-systems approach to patient management and will be expected to exercise a high degree of professional autonomy, particularly in relation to complex situations. By demonstrating an advanced level of clinical reasoning and decision-making, the NTC will make critical judgements that require a high level of understanding of the ethical and moral aspects of clinical practice.

A key element of expert clinical practice is to promote best practice through the synthesis and integration of research into practice. By taking a lead role in the development of protocols and pathways, the NTC will be able to facilitate the learning culture within the organisation or service. Furthermore, information and advances and or evaluations in practice can be cascaded through the organisation.

Professional leadership and consultancy

NTC roles all carry a significant professional leadership function. This includes providing leadership and clinical supervision to interprofessional teams crossing organisational and professional boundaries within patient care journeys. The requirement of the post-holders is to motivate and inspire others to advance practice and improve quality of care. Having the leadership skills to act as an agent of change is crucial to developing more innovative practices. This may involve challenging existing structures within organisations. The role of leadership will span across disciplines at a national and international level and locally within the employing organisation, reaffirming the points made in Figure 2.3.

Research and development

NTCs will have a key role in ensuring that patient services are high quality and based on the best evidence. They will lead and collaborate within their field to ensure the implementation and development of protocol-led services. They will co-ordinate and implement research projects incorporating inputs from a variety of disciplines, as well as identify gaps in the existing evidence base. A key role will be ensuring that new services are evaluated, which may lead to changes both within the organisation and more widely across the country. Working with higher education institutions to establish joint research partnerships will enhance the evidence base and give credence to new service designs. A role in monitoring clinical effectiveness through audit and research will ensure that clinical outcomes are evaluated and action plans are clearly identified and realised.

Education, training and development

The key function of the NTC in this delivery area is to promote and facilitate the development of a learning culture. This may be through acting as a role model or providing training and support to enable others to advance their skills at a range of levels. The NTC may have a role as a supervisor, mentor or educator and will establish links with institutes of higher education. Some NTCs will have roles in conjunction with higher education to plan, shape and deliver educational policies for both under- and postgraduate practitioners linked clearly to the relevant clinical speciality.

Interprofessional attributes

The broader concepts of nursing and therapy do not always fit well into current individual work patterns. The diversity of roles within the specialities to which NTCs are appointed also demand that experience, skills or actions provide a cross-functional purpose. Some of these cross-functional attributes, derived from a systematic review of past and current job descriptions, are outlined in Figure 3.2.

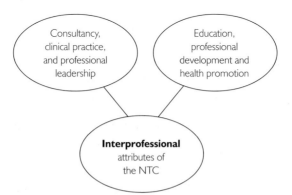

Figure 3.2 Interprofessional attributes of the NTC

Consultancy, clinical practice and professional leadership

As a consultant and expert clinical practitioner, the NTC is expected to provide direct care, advice management, leadership and supervision in high-quality patient focused services. This will determine evidenced-based therapeutic programmes of care to improve health outcomes and will lead to the development of collaborative integrated care pathways to provide streamlined, high-quality services for patients. The development of nurse/therapist-led protocols to provide diagnosis and treatment, and plan further management, may also be integral to this role.

Providing leadership to the nurse/therapist team in Trust-wide services and networking across organisational boundaries is part of the NTC's commitment to influence health care delivery positively within primary, secondary and tertiary care. The commitment actively to disseminate contributions to practice development by publishing and sharing good practice will further enhance the outcomes of NTC roles.

Education, professional development and health promotion

A major commitment may be expected of the NTC in the field of teaching, both locally and nationally, and may involve taking a lead role in training nurses and therapists within the specialities.

It may also involve the development of specific patient information literature and health promotion campaigns. Promotion of the service locally, nationally and internationally will be encouraged as NTCs submit publications to journals and conferences, and undertake external lectures at conferences and study days.

Personal attributes of the NTC

It is important for organisations who wish to appoint NTCs to think through the ideal personal specification and then place this within the reality of the candidates available. A personal specification that is set at too high a standard is likely to exclude some individuals who have the potential to perform very well in such a position. A personal specification that is set too low will lead to the appointment of an individual who may be too inexperienced and will require a greater investment in order to be successful in this position. Such an individual is likely to struggle to feel any sense of personal achievement, which, even in the more straightforward traditional appointments, can be difficult.

First-generation appointees may require greater support from institutions as they explore and establish their posts, often in the face of criticism from colleagues. In the early years, these appointees may not have positive role models to follow or opportunities to learn from their predecessors. A personal specification that identifies the personal attributes encapsulating the vision of the post should include some key features, identified in Figure 3.3.

Qualification requirements for a NTC
First-level registration
No matter what the discipline, all NTC posts require a formal recognition that the applicant be registered with both the professional governing body and the appropriate regulatory authority.

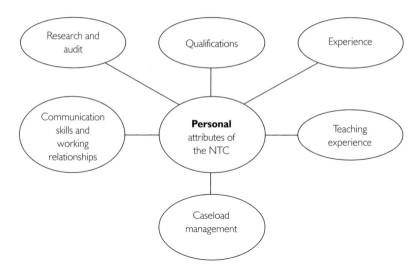

Figure 3.3   Personal attributes of the NTC

Relevant specialist postregistration qualifications
Many NTC posts require the applicant to hold some form of postregistration certification that is appropriate to the specialist area of practice. Where the posts include investigative procedures or surgical techniques, specific training courses will be stated as a minimum requirement. Some examples of these may include minor surgery, musculoskeletal therapy/rehabilitation and counselling certification.

Attainment of, or being within 1 year of completing, a relevant Master's qualification
The seniority of the NTC post demands that the applicant be able to demonstrate a high level of academic acumen. The initial advertisements placed a Master's qualification as a minimum standard, higher doctoral learning being viewed as an opportunity for further personal development as this had been proposed in the 'skills escalator' thinking. The realisation, however, that this could lessen the initial number of suitable candidates for nursing consultant posts forced a change in this standard.

Although the acquisition of a Master's followed by a doctoral qualification remains a long-term objective, the main thrust has been to concentrate on recruiting a sufficient number of individuals who have the potential to perform well in consultant posts. Emphasis is now being placed on the fact that there will be a future requirement to achieve at least a Master's degree qualification. The personal specification requirements have therefore been realigned and, as such, this level of qualification is currently considered to be a 'desirable requirement', with the understanding that it will become mandatory in the future.

Relevant experience
It appears from the job descriptions that we reviewed that there is a recommendation for NTCs to have a minimum of 10 years postregistration

experience, five of which must be recently within the speciality at a senior level. Although there appears to be wide variation in the duration of required postregistration experience, the consensus is that the individuals should be able to demonstrate that they have practised as professionals for a sufficient time in a registered capacity. This is so that they are well versed in the operation of the health service and the clinical issues that may arise during the course of their duties. There is frequently a lack of clarity over this issue as many personal specifications only mention five years in a senior position without being specific about what roles or responsibilities this may entail.

The knowledge to establish nursing and multidisciplinary audit and research

One of the four key delivery areas for the NTC is research and evaluation. The need for audit is therefore essential if the posts are to be able to demonstrate effectiveness as well as fitting in with the clinical governance agenda. Research projects should be based within practice and may well be evaluating new techniques, technology or services. They may well be interprofessional and closely aligned to the targets set in the modernisation agenda.

Teaching experience

It has been suggested that the NTC should have the knowledge to establish programmes of education within the workforce.

Working with local higher education establishments will be helpful. Academic staff will provide assistance with module construction, academic accreditation and administration when developing new or updated education programmes. This university accreditation is important to assist with personal development objectives for staff and to raise the profile of clinical departments and services.

It may be that modules are developed in the form of continued professional development programmes such as short courses or study days, or as part of a work-based Master's or Doctorate-level programme. As work-based learning is now being accepted as worthy of both academic and clinical credibility, the NTC will be in a position to bring expert knowledge to writing groups developing new curricula and helping to ensure that practice becomes more evidence-based.

Caseload management

Experience in developing and managing programmes of care is essential. The essence of a consultant is the acceptance of the responsibility for a patient caseload. Each patient requires a clinical management plan that can range from the straightforward to the complex.

The NTC will need to identify the shifting boundaries of patient care so that referrals can be made or received for a caseload that is appropriate to the individual's skill levels or professional responsibility. Many of the programmes of care will be obvious from established pathways and protocols, but as practice parameters shift, or new evidence comes to recommend changes in management, the NTC will need to be confident in developing innovation in practice and involving the wider interdisciplinary team.

Communication skills and working relationships

Good communication skills are essential if the individual is to be successful. The interagency involvement of the NTC will be a key feature of this post. Agencies may include individuals and departments within local institutions, for example nursing teams, medical teams, directors of services and Trust boards. There are also a wide range of contacts external to the larger institutions that are important in local health and social care. These include Primary Care Trusts, community teams, specialist colleagues and members of the Workforce Development Confederation and the Strategic Health Authority. Effective communication requires that the NTC strives to find common ground at a strategic level on which to base the foundations of effective practice and development. In summary, it appears, through examining current job descriptions, that the NTC post-holder will have three key attributes:

- personal – is a self-starter able to inspire and lead others
- professional – can demonstrate expert professional practice and initiate service developments
- interprofessional – is a good communicator able to develop a wide range of working relationships.

These are illustrated in Figure 3.4.

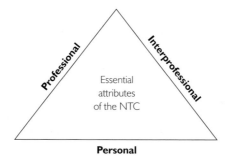

Figure 3.4 The emerging attributes of the NTC: findings from a role analysis

Activity 3.2 *Feedback*

The essential attributes of the NTC

It is evident from the information contained within this chapter that there are three key elements to the essential attributes – personal, professional and interprofessional. Implicit in and essential to these attributes are the qualifications, knowledge, skills and levels of clinical experience that the NTC will require to perform and evaluate the post.

PRESENTING THE KEY ATTRIBUTES THROUGH A REVIEW OF JOB DESCRIPTIONS AND PERSONAL SPECIFICATIONS

The following section details an example of a personal specification (Table 3.1) and a number of job descriptions (Boxes 3.3–3.6) based on the findings of a role analysis of some current NTC posts. It is by no means a complete set of personal specification requirements but a summary of those which appear most often and seem key to the development of the role.

Overall, there is a close consensus of agreement from the job descriptions that we reviewed, and similar categories were identified. We have included a range of tables to demonstrate that job descriptions are currently either based quite obviously on the four key roles or take a more wider remit and use broader categories such as skills, experience and knowledge.

The following are extracts from a selection of job descriptions and personal specifications from general nursing, mental health nursing and allied health profession posts across the United Kingdom. What is apparent from these job specifications is that no matter what speciality the vacancy is in, there is little direction on the specific remit of what constitutes 'expert clinical practice'.

Personal specification

Table 3.1   Example of a personal specification for the NTC

	Essential	Desirable
Qualifications/education	Professional registration Master's level (or undertaking current study) Accreditation in the area of specialist practice Teaching courses (e.g. English National Board Certificate 998, or City and Guilds 730 Certificate, Practice Educators course)	Research qualification Higher teaching qualification (e.g. Postgraduate Diploma in Education)
Skills/abilities	Skilled therapeutic specialist Evidence of clinical examination and history taking skills Good written and verbal communication skills Ability to work efficiently under pressure Teaching skills appropriate to the area of specialist practice Effective time management skills Ability to work within and motivate a team	Ability to use PC and associated software
Experience	Five years postregistration experience in the specialist field at a senior level Experience of developing extended/expanded policies/protocols Experience in audit Track record of innovation Change management experience Has demonstrated involvement in research and practice development	Computer literacy Understanding of the professional research agenda
Knowledge	Has demonstrated knowledge of the specialist field at an expert level Knowledge of relevant pharmacological practice	Has published material Has lectured at local/national conferences

	Essential	Desirable
	A clear understanding of recent NHS reforms and national guidelines	
	Understanding of the research process	
	Understanding of the clinical governance framework	
Disposition	Enthusiastic, highly motivated	Dynamic
	A willingness to accept responsibility while providing clinical leadership to a committed team	Self-assured
	Trustworthy	
	Flexible working approach	
	Self-motivated	
	Team player	
	Approachable manner	
	Sense of humour	

Box 3.3   Example of a job description – adult mental health

NURSE CONSULTANT ADULT MENTAL HEALTH SERVICE AIMS AND OBJECTIVES

The future aims and objectives within Adult Mental Health are those outlined within the National Service Framework for Mental Health. They include:

- access to single-sex accommodation in hospital
- a reduction in the psychiatric emergency readmission rate
- experience of service users/carers in the planning, development and evaluation of services
- a reduction in bed occupancy rates
- a reduction in suicide rates
- 24 hour access to services.

The locality is currently in the process of significant modernisation of its main acute inpatient area, which will create an improved environment structurally and see the development of a High Dependency Unit. Alongside changes in the actual physical environment changes are innovative and exciting changes planned/in planning stage to improve and develop care pathways and processes for service users, and enhanced clinical roles/leadership for staff.

Role of the Nurse Consultant

It is against this background that the role of Nurse Consultant Adult Mental Health is being proposed. Working primarily within the acute psychiatric inpatient facilities, the post-holder will also link into the Community Mental Health Teams. This, it is envisaged, will focus on the opportunities to develop skills and practices into the acute area of psychiatric nursing care and treatment. Utilisation of key therapies, including Psychosocial Interventions

(PSI) and Cognitive Behavioural Therapies (CBT), underpinned by the continued development of multidisciplinary working, joint assessment and the evolving integration of the Care Programme Approach and Care Management, will provide a firm base for these developments and changes to take place. Interface into the newer services of Assertive Outreach and Home Treatment services further enhances the comprehensive range of opportunities for proactive working.

In achieving this role, the Nurse Consultant will fulfil the key functions as outlined in HSC/1999/217 (Department of Health, 1999b), namely:

- expert clinical practice
- professional leadership and consultancy function
- education, training and development function
- research and development.

Key working relationships
Users and carers
The Trust is committed to the involvement of, listening to and acting upon the views and opinions of users and carers. As a 'Supporter' of the 'Breakthrough' organisation, which strives to inform and work with user/advocacy groups to campaign for changes in Mental Health Services, strong local groups exist throughout the locality. It is seen as an integral part of the Nurse Consultant's role to integrate these viewpoints into nursing activities.

Voluntary sector
Across the locality, some services are provided by voluntary sector organisations and link closely with statutory providers. Again, it is vital that the Nurse Consultant role integrates this viewpoint and input from non-statutory sector.

Strong links exist with several academic institutions, in particular the local university. An Honorary Lecturer's post for the Nurse Consultant will enable input into basic and postbasic training. Research facilities will also be available.

The Trust has also developed a strategic approach to training and education in respect of PSI. This has included the development of a PSI Training and Education Officer to link with academic institutions in the development of relevant academic courses. Awareness-raising seminars and a Special Interest Group maintain the momentum of this important evidence-based model of care delivery. It is the expectation that the Nurse Consultant will play a part in the implementation of this strategy.

Centre for Mental Health
Centre for Mental Health is part of group regional centre for mental health. The Trust is committed to this group and regularly participates in studies and workshops to drive forward the Mental Health agenda.

Nurse Advisory Group

A central Nurse Advisory Group exists with specialist subgroups in the areas of Practice Development, Education and Training, and Research and Development. Links into this group in a consultative and advisory capacity will be expected, plus other groups as required. These may include Clinical Governance and the NSF Local Implementation Teams Mental Health Act Steering Group.

A regional, national and international profile will further assist in promoting practice in Adult Mental Health. It is expected that links with organisations such as the National Institute for Clinical Excellence (NICE) and the Centre for Health Improvements (CHI) would be maintained.

Funding

Funding for the development of this post has been secured within the Trust's budgets in line with HSC 1999/217 (Department of Health, 1999b) for a salary circa £28,000–42,000.

Box 3.4   Example of a job description – emergency care

NURSE CONSULTANT IN EMERGENCY CARE

1 Introduction

Establishing a Nurse Consultant post within the Accident & Emergency setting will support the achievement of NHS priorities in relation to meeting demands for prompt and effective services and the achievement of targets within the National Service Framework for Coronary Heart Disease.

The post-holder will develop the concept of Clinical Governance with an element of practical research as well as integrating research findings into practice. He/she will lead the Clinical Governance agenda in relation to nursing within the directorate.

2 Proposal

2.1 The Nurse Consultant post will have a number of dimensions that together improve the overall service and clinical practices offered to patients in the Accident & Emergency Directorate. Key functions will include:

- the development and implementation of a nursing model of care, specific to Accident & Emergency nursing
- providing expert direct clinical care to patients within agreed protocols; providing advice and support to colleagues where standard protocols do not apply
- the training and education of staff, particularly in relation to thrombolysis and the management of the acute myocardial infarction
- leading research, evaluation and audit

- co-ordinating and supervising nursing research activities within the Directorate
- taking responsibility for organising and ensuring that the Clinical Governance framework is embedded into the ethos of the Accident & Emergency nursing
- identifying, measuring and monitoring key critical outcomes for patients, e.g. acute myocardial infarction, door-to-needle times
- the standardisation of best practice by implementing evidence-based nursing care within the two hospitals of this newly merged Trust.

2.2 The role will be focused on the development of Accident & Emergency care. Essential elements of the role include:
- the training, education and ongoing development of skills within the Accident & Emergency department
- ensuring the delivery of a quality service
- monitoring and maintaining standards of care delivered.

3 Assessment of service needs

3.1 There are currently 42,000 new patients presenting to the Accident & Emergency department, and these are continuing to increase with pressure for access to acute medical beds.

3.2 The launch of the National Service Framework for Coronary Heart Disease introduces unique challenges in meeting call-to-needle times, with a target of 20 minutes for the delivery of thrombolysis from the call for help; this necessitates early diagnosis and treatment.

3.3 Increasing pressure on beds within acute medicine as a consequence of Emergency pressures has reflected on the number of acutely ill patients being referred to the Accident & Emergency department: during 2000; a 75% increase in patients being treated in the resuscitation facilities has been noted.

4 Re-engineering Accident & Emergency services

4.1 The whole process of treatment within the Accident & Emergency department is regularly reviewed to ensure that there is an effective use of resources and that patients are admitted and discharged appropriately.

4.2 The Emergency Nurse Consultant will complement and support further development of the nurse's role in relation to Accident & Emergency nursing. This will encompass areas such as clinical protocols, guidelines in relation to nurse-led care provision, and evaluation of the effect of changes through audit, research and outcome indicators.

4.3 As the role evolves, the Emergency Nurse Consultant will stretch the boundaries of practice innovation, defining and developing new roles within nurse-led care and advancing professional practice to benefit patients, for example in nurse-led resuscitation in the cardiac arrest situation.

4.4 Quality is now at the heart of the NHS service delivery, and there is an imperative for all professionals to ensure that services are patient focused and practices evidence based. The Emergency Nurse Consultant will facilitate this by leading the research and clinical governance agenda for the directorate.

5 Dimensions of the post

The main aims of the post are centred around:

- an expert clinical practice function
- a professional leadership and consultancy function
- an education, training and development function
- a practice and service development, research and evaluation function.

The above functions contribute to the development of a practitioner whose base is firmly placed in clinical practice.

5.1 Expert clinical practice function

The Nurse Consultant will be an expert in the field of Accident & Emergency nursing and have a wide experience of knowledge and expertise of policy, practice and research pertaining to the acutely ill patient.

The post-holder will be an essential link in the multidisciplinary team. The Emergency Nurse Consultant will accept responsibility for clinical activity, providing a high degree of professional autonomy, and making critical judgements where precedence does not exist, without recourse to others to satisfy the expectations and demands of the job.

The post-holder will exercise a high degree of personal professional autonomy and make critical judgements of the highest order. He/she will have the ability to make decisions where precedents do not exist, without recourse to others, and to advise and support colleagues where standard protocols do not exist.

5.2 Professional leadership function

The Emergency Nurse Consultant will be instrumental in leading and developing a specific nursing team in promoting best practice standards within nurse-led care.

The post-holder will be expected to improve standards and quality and to develop nurse-led professional practice within the Accident & Emergency care setting. Developing and promoting best practice and setting standards will be a key component of the role.

The Emergency Nurse Consultant will have a key role in providing expert advice to others, both internally and externally to the Accident & Emergency department; this will include services such as primary care and NHS Direct. This will include contributing to longer-term strategic planning for Accident & Emergency services as well as delivering structured and ad hoc support to the team.

The individual will be expected to share their expertise, acting as a resource for others and providing support within and outside the organisation.

5.3 Education, training and development

The Emergency Nurse Consultant will contribute to internal and external training and development. A key role will be the sharing of good practice and the dissemination of information within the field of Accident & Emergency, both locally and nationally.

Specifically, he/she will be responsible for the development of education programmes for the nursing body within the Trust, the evaluation of such programmes and the updating and ongoing advanced professional development of individuals within the Directorate.

The Emergency Nurse Consultant will play a key role in helping to integrate theory with practice and will develop and sustain productive partnerships with local universities.

5.4 Practice and service developments

Developments in Accident & Emergency service delivery and practice will be the key to the success of the Emergency Nurse Consultant, and the individual will require extensive knowledge of the complexities of practice development activities.

Key responsibilities will be the promotion of evidence-based practice, setting, monitoring and auditing standards relating to nurse-led Accident & Emergency practice, and identifying and promoting measures to define, evaluate and secure quality improvement.

The post-holder will be expected to apply research to practice and develop the skills of others in order to facilitate the research process.

Box 3.5 Example of job description – consultant physiotherapist

Job Title:	Consultant Physiotherapist
Grade:	Consultant Therapist
Department:	Therapies Directorate
Division:	Clinical Support Services

Reporting relationships

Accountable to:	Head of Division for work in musculoskeletal clinics
	Clinical Director for Therapies for work within physiotherapy
Responsible to:	Lead Consultant for work in musculoskeletal clinics
	Clinical Director for Therapies for work within physiotherapy
	Key relationships: Clinical Directors, Clinicians, Therapists, other Allied Health

	Professional (AHP) staff, Nursing Staff, Nurse Consultants, University Staff
Professionally accountable to:	Clinical Director for Therapies

Role summary

The Consultant Therapist in Musculoskeletal Disease will provide hands-on treatment within a defined clinical area, along with Consultant duties within the musculoskeletal clinics. He or she will demonstrate expert knowledge and work closely alongside consultant medical colleagues. He or she will also develop individuals within the Musculoskeletal Physiotherapy Team and demonstrate an improved provision of effective clinical interventions. He or she will be expected to take a leading role in the musculoskeletal clinics, delivering expert assessments within that environment, and will also have a key role in crossing organisational and professional boundaries, linking together interventions along the care pathway. The post-holder will play a key role in identifying training needs and maximising development opportunities for staff within the Musculoskeletal Therapies Team. The overall aim of the post is to ensure that patients are assessed and treated effectively, along with developing the role of practitioners working within the Musculoskeletal Team.

Main duties and responsibilities

1. Expert clinical practice
1.1 To provide expert clinical skill and advanced knowledge.
1.2 To act in an educational capacity for postgraduate staff, and to advise and teach on the undergraduate course.
1.3 To liaise with all members of the multidisciplinary teams.
1.4 To provide a developmental role for all extended role practitioners within the Musculoskeletal Team.
1.5 To support and advise staff throughout the Trust on musculoskeletal diseases issues.
1.6 To develop and implement innovations in improvements in clinical practice.
1.7 To lead in the development of musculoskeletal clinical standards.

2. Professional leadership and consultancy
2.1 To provide clinical leadership for all AHP staff working in the area of musculoskeletal disease.
2.2 To contribute to the regional/national agenda.
2.3 To lead on the distribution and publication of research.
2.4 To lead on the promotion and development of best clinical evidence.
2.5 To contribute to the development of senior physiotherapists.

3. Education, training and development
3.1 To work in partnership with the local university, contributing to the undergraduate curriculum and postgraduate teaching.

3.2 To participate in regional networks and push forward the education and development of staff.

3.3 To work with the wider multidisciplinary team in training events.

4. Practice and service development, research and evaluation

4.1 To contribute to the Musculoskeletal Physiotherapy Service by a critical analysis of skill mix.

4.2 To work with stakeholders to develop practice within varied settings.

4.3 To develop the practice of non-medical practitioners functioning in a consultancy capacity.

4.4 To lead on research and development within the Musculoskeletal Team and to collaborate with research in the Locomotor Division.

4.5 To act as an assessor and advisor for postgraduate dissertations and assignments.

4.6 To support other agencies in the application of research-finding.

4.7 To take part in and develop a thorough evaluation of the role of Consultant Therapist within the musculoskeletal clinics.

5. Health and safety

5.1 To take reasonable care for their own health and safety and that of any other person who may be affected by their acts or omissions at work.

5.2 To co-operate with the Hospital NHS Trust in ensuring that statutory regulations, codes of practice, local policies and departmental health and safety rules are adhered to.

6. Professional development

6.1 To take every reasonable opportunity to maintain and improve their professional knowledge and competence.

6.2 To participate in personal objective-setting and review, including the creation of a personal development plan.

7. Confidentiality

7.1 To ensure that confidentiality is maintained at all times in conjunction with the Trust's Confidentiality Policy.

This job description is *not* exhaustive and is only intended to be a guide to the principal duties and responsibilities of the post. It may be amended at any time with the agreement of the post-holder and line manager.

Box 3.6 Example of job description – rehabilitative care

Title of post:	Nurse Consultant Post in Rehabilitative Care
Department:	Directorate of Orthopaedics
Professionally accountable to:	Director of Nursing
Managerially accountable to:	Clinical Director (Orthopaedics) 1

1 Role summary

- The post will have a key strategic function within the rehabilitative and intermediate services and a specific clinical function within the Orthopaedic Directorate directed towards those patients recovering from trauma. The post-holder will have an important role in integrating nursing policy, education, practice development and research relevant to patients receiving rehabilitative care within all clinical settings.
- To provide professional and clinical leadership to all nurses involved in rehabilitative care within all care settings, empowering staff to make a difference.
- To have a lead role in the development of an infrastructure that enables the introduction of evidence-based protocols and guidelines to be disseminated and implemented within the Trust.
- To lead and develop a new model of inpatient and community rehabilitation/intermediate care services, including the establishment of the Nurse Consultant's autonomous practice and leadership role.
- To lead and develop integrated multidisciplinary/agency pathways of care covering a range of treatment and care options for inpatient, intermediate and community care, ensuring an effective transition between subsequent phases of care and treatment.
- To lead the development of protocols and criteria for accessing, and discharging from, specific pathways.
- To maintain a patient caseload providing expert care, advice and counselling to patients and carers outwith protocols without recourse to others.
- To forge and maintain critical alliances with social services and the private and voluntary sectors who currently have, or who have the potential to contribute to, the care of this client group.
- To lead the development of outcome indicators for the rehabilitation service.
- To demonstrate an increase in patient satisfaction by providing a patient/carer-centred approach to practice incorporating the user perspective in future service developments.
- To demonstrate an improvement in patient outcomes, service and quality by developing a range of multidisciplinary/multiagency indicators

benchmarked against national and international standards, and to implement changes aimed at achieving best practice.
- To contribute to reduced pressure on acute beds and extended or inappropriate stays in rehabilitative beds.

2 Main duties and responsibilities

2.1 Practice function

The post-holder will spend at least 50% of their time in clinical practice and will require expert clinical skills and knowledge in the clinical speciality and rehabilitation. These skills will include advanced clinical examination and assessment skills.

The post-holder will manage a caseload and assess, plan, deliver and evaluate the nursing interventions offered to this group in any care setting (including a key role within the private sector). He/she will ensure a clear coherent application of evidence-based nursing care, which is integrated into, and complementary to, the care offered by other members of the multidisciplinary/multiagency team. The post-holder will have the ability and autonomy to make decisions where precedents do not exist, without recourse to others, and to advise and support colleagues where standard protocols do not apply.

The post-holder will develop and lead integrated pathways of care involving all agencies and monitor and evaluate their application and effectiveness in any care setting, with the aim of maximising patients' health potential or minimising the effects of ill-health or disability.

The post-holder will need to decide how the appropriateness of alternative rehabilitative packages/pathways will be decided at the beginning of the care episode facilitated by agreed, shared protocols. These protocols will include the application of indicators, which will direct patients on to appropriate rehabilitative pathways prior to any surgical intervention. Thereafter, the Nurse Consultant will be autonomous in leading the rehabilitation phase by identifying which pathway/package of care is most appropriate for the individual in both inpatient and community settings by working across existing organisational and agency boundaries.

The post-holder will develop and agree protocols that will enable him/her to:

- accept direct referrals
- develop nurse-led clinics
- prescribe investigatory procedures and refer on to other specialist services
- admit into acute and community care
- make direct referrals to other professionals with due regard to the multipathological nature of this client group.

Summary of clinical activities
- Accepting direct referrals for access into specific care pathways that integrate both health and social care needs.

- Prescribing and initiating care packages in both community and acute settings, with the autonomy to make referrals to any other professional involved in the care process.
- Ensuring that all interventions are prebooked before the initial acute surgical phase is complete, within both acute and community settings.
- Reviewing patients and evaluating their progress at specific intervals.
- Monitoring the care package and taking autonomous action as required.
- Discharging from rehabilitative care or into the care of other professionals if multipathology is present.
- Evaluating the whole episode of care.

2.2 Leadership and consultancy function

To provide professional and clinical leadership to all nurses working within the rehabilitative services, including the establishment of effective mechanisms for clinical supervision.

The post-holder will be a key driver in service developments in rehabilitative and intermediate care that will be based on research evidence and the needs of the local population, and which cross traditional organisational boundaries within both hospital and community settings. To facilitate this, the post-holder will work in close collaboration with clinical directors, service managers, Primary Care Groups/Trusts, Social Services, the private sector, etc. and be an active member of the Professional Nursing and Midwifery Advisory Group and the Clinical Policy Board. He/she will create and sustain effective working relationships with all agencies involved in the provision of rehabilitative/ intermediate care at both a strategic and an operational level.

The post-holder will have a specific role related to his/her area of clinical practice in both acute and community settings and will act as a referral point for nursing and other related disciplines. He/she will act as an internal and external consultant for all disciplines regarding the availability and appropriateness of rehabilitative care. In addition, he/she will offer advice to, and forge and sustain new alliances with, other agencies involved in the provision of services in order to increase or improve their capacity to care effectively for this client group.

The post-holder will play a lead role for clinical governance in the Directorate, reviewing policies, protocols and guidelines relating to rehabilitative and intermediate care.

2.3 Education, training and development function

The post-holder will develop and participate in learning programmes for all staff, within all settings and organisations that support professional and personal development. A major aim of such activity will be to increase the ability of all in rehabilitative skills, thereby reducing the demand on the specialist services. Additionally, primary prevention will be a key focus of this educational provision, linking in with the priorities of the Health Improvement Programmes.

The post-holder will establish, maintain and foster genuine relationships with higher educational institutions. He/she will assist universities and other bodies in evaluating existing educational provision and the commissioning of new or amended courses. The post-holder will identify new multidisciplinary and multiagency learning and development opportunities, and liaise with both internal and external providers to develop and implement such courses.

The post-holder will raise the profile of rehabilitative and intermediate care training and development in the Trust's individual development planning processes, thereby ensuring that Directorates address training and development in relation to rehabilitative/intermediate care in their business plans.

Through appropriate education, training and development, the post-holder will support nursing staff and others in implementating national standards relating to rehabilitative/intermediate care.

2.4 Practice and service development, research and evaluation function
The post-holder will promote and demonstrate research-based practice, initiating research projects and supporting staff involved in research. He/she will act as an internal and external consultant advising on appropriate practice and service developments based upon the evidence available and local health population needs (as expressed through local Health Improvement Programmes), which meet local, regional and national strategies/priorities.

In collaboration with other professional leads and other agencies (including the private sector), the post-holder will ensure that any national frameworks for the delivery of rehabilitative/intermediate care services are implemented.

The post-holder will work with local universities and regional and national agencies to establish partnerships to carry out, participate in, or commission research within the field of rehabilitative/intermediate care, and will contribute to the academic arena through clinical teaching, research, writing for publication and conference presentations.

He/she will ensure his/her own continuous professional development through embracing the principles of lifelong learning to Master's level and above, and develop and maintain local, regional and national frameworks to promote peer support and facilitate clinical supervision.

The post-holder will constantly monitor and evaluate the achievement of explicit outcome indicators for the rehabilitation service, and lead and collaborate with the multidisciplinary/multiagency team regarding any changes in service delivery or practice suggested by the results. He/she will identify appropriate changes in service provision, which will ensure that the care and treatment of individuals are provided in the most appropriate setting, thereby enhancing the utilisation of current services in both community and acute settings.

In summary, the personal specification and job descriptions above reinforce the emerging attributes of the NTC and demonstrate a high level of personal and professional expertise.

This debate is covered in Chapter 1.

CONCLUSION

The role of the NTC is still in its infancy. For those who have been in post for two or more years, there is still much work to be done with the evolution of the role. Future objectives for NTCs will depend on a multitude of variables that are affected by the personal qualities of the post-holders and their backgrounds, the acceptance of the position within the institutions and the refinements of the job descriptions for each post. There is no right way to 'do' the NTC role, but equally there is no wrong way. For some, the research opportunities will be key from the outset. For others, this will be developmental and considered to be part of their professional development. The same can be said of the provision of education.

Putting the NTC post together requires support, resources and opportunity. Opportunities arise through applying what you know and seeking out what you don't know. The ongoing political drivers will to a certain extent dictate what opportunities are yet to come. The major influences on my role have been the targets of the National Service Frameworks (NSFs) and the Reforming Emergency Care programme, but the full impact of the implementation of the European Working Time Directives has yet to be realised. Reforms will present the NHS with further opportunities for NTCs to become embedded in health care and be widely accepted as a necessity and an asset in the provision of a modern service.

SUMMARY OF KEY POINTS

- The four key roles of the NTC are those of expert clinical practice; professional leadership and consultancy; education, training and development; and research and development.
- The role analysis carried out of current job descriptions and feedback from current post-holders has demonstrated that the NTC post has three key attributes – personal, professional and interprofessional.
- Contained within these three elements are subattributes associated with having essential qualifications, knowledge, skills and levels of clinical experience to perform and evaluate the post efficiently and effectively.
- To understand the role of the NTC within your own organisation, we would strongly recommend that you carry out a 'role analysis' by reviewing your job description and your personal specification within your own organisation; you can enlist the support of another NTC for this. This may enable you to understand the scope and context of your post within the workplace.

CASE STUDY 3.1 **A PRACTICAL APPROACH HIGHLIGHTING THE ESSENTIAL ATTRIBUTES OF THE NTC THROUGH PERSONAL REFLECTIONS ON THE ROLE OF THE NURSE CONSULTANT**

J Campbell Nurse Consultant, Emergency Care.

Introduction

The purpose of this section is to provide an open and honest account of my experiences as a Nurse Consultant. These reflections will hopefully highlight the complexities that are involved in this role. While I am aware that each post is individual, I feel confident, from the clinical supervision sessions that I attend, that the examples here have also been experienced by other Nurse Consultants. I have tried to concentrate on the major issues that demonstrate what attributes I have needed in order to function, and point out that the examples are not an exhaustive list! After each section, the activity boxes invite you to think about the essential attributes that are required for each of the four key functions.

Background

The development of the Nurse Consultant in emergency care was founded on the need to achieve the targets set out in the NSF for coronary heart disease (CHD) (DoH, 2000c). The relevant issues were to work towards the achievement of the targets for the provision of thrombolysis for patients suffering an acute myocardial infarction (AMI), in particular developing a thrombolysis service in the Accident & Emergency department. Although this example covers the role of a Nurse Consultant, the context may also be relevant to other Consultant posts.

For many hospitals, coronary care units proliferated in the 1960s and 70s to provide the monitoring and early recognition of lethal arrhythmias that occurred following AMI. Few of these units were sited near Accident & Emergency departments or had ground-floor access. From the 1980s, increasing importance has been placed on the use of thrombolytic agents to facilitate the reperfusion of myocardial tissue. The NSF for CHD disseminated an understanding of the importance of early intervention using this treatment. The location of coronary care units away from direct ambulance access forced the adoption of a broader remit for ground-floor Accident & Emergency departments when planning and setting up thrombolysis services.

This has added to the increasing pressure on Accident & Emergency departments that have seen a rise in patient throughput. Locally, the nature of work for Accident & Emergency staff had focused on the management and treatment of both minor and major trauma. Recently, however, the extreme pressure on bed availability in medical admissions areas has necessitated a diversification of the role towards the management of medical emergencies without the volume of retraining that is required to prepare the staff adequately. The addition of the thrombolysis service to the workload of Accident & Emergency departments has put even more pressure on the already overstretched service, with little in the way of supportive resources.

Aims

The aims of the post include:

- the provision of expert direct clinical care to patients within agreed protocols, providing advice to colleagues where standard protocols do not apply
- the training and education of staff, particularly in relation to thrombolysis and the management of AMI
- leading research, evaluation and audit
- the standardisation of best practice by implementing evidence-based nursing care.

Reflection

Starting a new job in a new department is always a daunting prospect, and taking on a role that has never existed raises this level of apprehension. In addition, the implementation of the role of the Nurse Consultant has been perceived by many as an unknown political initiative, one carrying a high price tag in comparison to other nursing posts. Attitudes towards the concept of Nurse Consultant have varied from being aggressively against it to a position of apathy fuelled by lack of understanding. Only a very few people have had a positive attitude towards exploring how the concept could be developed and applied to a service that was anticipating shortfalls in all disciplines of staff, not least junior medical staff.

Induction to the post

I felt that it was important, in the initial months of the appointment, to become a visible member of the team, and much of my time was spent gaining experience in the Accident & Emergency department, contributing to the care of patients whom I felt comfortable managing and observing the work involved for patients with problems of which I had little experience. This induction period was also used to meet a number of key players within, or in key positions related to, the organisation and those with whom establishing a relationship was important for future service development. Having joined the Trust just before being appointed to the Nurse Consultant role was an asset as many internal relationships had already been established. This helped to reduce the duration of induction. The induction period was important as this confirmed what I thought were the opportunities for the post.

Expert clinical practice

Performing a direct hands-on role providing thrombolysis for a limited number of patients who require it is neither an efficient use of a resource nor a way to provide a sufficient clinical workload on a day-to-day basis. The greater problem for the

---

Box 3.7   Proposed remit for the Nurse Consultant in emergency care based on the job
description and assessment of local need management of chest pain

- Interface between hospital and ambulance
- Interface between hospital & GPs
- Provision of care for patients with chest pain
- Interface between agencies providing education to public
- Adoption and promotion of evidence-based practice

Accident & Emergency department is, however, those patients who present with
non-specific chest pain who have no access to follow-up review. Diversification of the
role was identified very early on as a necessity. The expansion of the Rapid Access
Chest Pain Clinic (RACPC) to include patients who presented to Accident &
Emergency rather than their GP gave an opportunity to provide one-to-one expert
clinical care. This also allowed a regular clinical session that could fit into a timetable
that would continue to include the assessment of patients presenting acutely. The
assessment and treatment of patients was not restricted to the Accident &
Emergency department alone. The Nurse Consultant position facilitated the
introduction of acute chest pain assessment in any area so that patients with new-
onset chest pain could be swiftly assessed and early treatment initiated in a co-
ordinated manner.

Box 3.8   Summary of key function: expert clinical practice

- Assessment and treatment of patients with chest pain
  - Accident & Emergency
  - Coronary care unit
  - Medical assessment unit
  - Wards
- RACPC

Practice and service development, research and evaluation

The alignment of this role to the NSF for CHD provided the standards against which
performance would be audited. This was not the focus *on* the role but more the focus
of the role. The door-to-needle time audit was well established; what my role has
offered is a central point of contact through which processes can be channelled. These
processes include the validation of cases to be included in the national audit project;
the review of those who are treated outside the target times; and the presentation of
audit reports to clinical and managerial staff with suggestions on how to improve
performance, together with the costings for new resources that are highlighted.

The introduction of a thrombolysis service to the Accident & Emergency department
was part of the NSF for CHD. Reviewing the local policies and producing simple flow

charts for the treatment of patients with AMI contributed to the development of this service. The development of a 24-hour nurse-led service for thrombolysis was considered as an option, and may still be potentially achievable, but it does not currently offer a cost-effective use of available resources.

Contributing to the local implementation team for the NSF put me in a position where I was seen as a key link into secondary care services in our locality. This introduced me to the ambulance service representatives, who requested that I assist with the implementation of 12-lead ECG transmission systems. I was now in a position to influence not only door-to-needle times, but also, in partnership with community services, call-to-needle times. This is a facilitatory position that helps the hospital to understand what the ambulance service is trying to achieve, and the ambulance service to understand how best the hospital can use its resources to optimise the impact of this initiative.

Involvement in the RACPC produced the opportunity not only to compare performance against NSF targets, but also to introduce the concept of holistic care to the clinic. There had been a chest pain service for some years, but until the NSF for CHD was published, there had been no targets against which this could be measured. We needed to address the target of all patients being seen within 14 days of the date of referral; this called for collaboration with local GPs and Primary Care Trusts. Developing a referral to the primary care CHD rehabilitation service proved more straightforward than had been expected as the community CHD nurses were more than willing to accept these new patients. This is perhaps the greatest quality improvement implemented to date. It also demonstrates that there can be good reasons to transpose nursing on to an area of medical practice, not for the sake of becoming a mini-medic but to implement a real improvement in patient care.

Box 3.9 Summary of key function: practice and service development, research and e valuation

- Audit of thrombolysis door-to-needle times
- Introduction of thrombolysis to Accident & Emergency
- Development of referral pathways to primary care CHD nurses for patients with newly diagnosed angina
- Evaluation of the RACPC service
- Development of a coronary angiography service
- Evaluation of the role of the Nurse Consultant

Education, training and development

Having had links with education for several years in my previous posts, part of which had been spent as a lecturer-practitioner acting between the Trust and the local university, addressing the education component of the NTC role was the least daunting for me. Maintaining the link with the university was important, partly because I needed to be able to identify with a part of my role that was familiar to me and in which I was confident that I could deliver a high standard of practice. In addition, this area provided an opportunity to promote the role of the NTC as something that a broader audience could recognise. From this has arisen a network of contacts that I have used for other aspects of the role or to help individuals who have come to me for further training or consultancy. The development of the Nurse Consultant role, and the pool of expertise from individuals with clinical credibility that this produced, was soon recognised and enthusiastically received by the university. Appointments to honorary lecturerships within the academic institutions were quick to follow the taking up of posts in the clinical areas. Involvement of the NTCs in the university continues to be appreciated as being mutually beneficial.

The teaching role and the development of training within the Trust contributed to contact with local nursing and medical teams. Delivering a variety of teaching sessions has helped to construct an image of a positive role model and, as with the role within the university, has helped to establish closer and more internal networks.

Speaking at conferences at a national level is expected, as it is in many NTC job descriptions. Through my involvement in nurse prescribing, I was asked to give a brief talk at a regional meeting to promote the role of nurse/pharmacist prescribing. Although this might not have been quite national level, it was certainly useful, not only in sharing my own experiences, but also in understanding some of the difficulties of this initiative that are experienced in other health care areas, as well as the opinions of Department of Health representatives.

On reflection, the key 'take-home message' that I gained in relation to my role was not connected with the subject of the day. Before I attended this conference, I still felt very much the novice consultant and believed that I was not involved at a high enough level that my involvement with nurse prescribing would meet what I believed to be a national-level standard. I was, however, very wrong. The lack of debate at any level with regard to experiences of implementing nurse prescribing as a practitioner has provided me with an opportunity to address the national stage, assuming that I am prepared to put in more effort to establish further networks or publish more material about this area. It is therefore down to me, and my levels of energy and motivation, to achieve this. I do not look at this as a failure as I am quite content with my efforts so far, and no one offering appraisal has criticised me for this. This is an opportunity to be achieved in future year(s') objectives.

The greatest resource for me as a Nurse Consultant has been using opportunities to integrate with other Nurse Consultants. Learning from and relating to other people's experiences helps me to appreciate that I am not the only person with a particular view point. Learning that different approaches have been employed to develop NTC roles gave me the confidence to feel that whichever way I chose to approach my role would be the right approach, and that it was important for me to feel comfortable with what I was doing. Clinical supervision groups and Nurse Consultant development groups have been essential for sharing these details and understanding what is contemporary in the political, service and academic arenas. Non-clinical personal development objectives identified from such meetings have often provided a basis from which more detailed learning could evolve.

Personal development for clinical objectives has been dependent on the opportunities that have arisen and on how the role has evolved. Some of these opportunities were easily identified from the remit that was originally proposed for this role; other development needs have been presented with the introduction of new initiatives. One example of this is independent nurse prescribing. This was judged to be ideally suited to the Nurse Consultant role with the prospect to expand to other disciplines as need dictated. It did, however, require that I attend the university for the statutory training and examination. Had this not been 'suggested', I would have overlooked what has been a good learning experience and an access to further extended nursing. I would also not have been able to establish some of the primary care networks that I now have and the involvement with other organisations.

Box 3.10   Summary of key function: education, training and development

- In-house training
  - Nursing technical and medical staff
  - Critical care network
- Honorary lecturer (university based)
  - Postregistration education
    Critical care core skills
    Clinical skills
    Interpretation of the ECG (new module for 2004)
  - Contribution to development of professional Doctorate
- National
  - Nurse prescribing workshop
- Continuing professional development
  - Nurse Consultant clinical supervision
  - Extended nurse prescribing
  - Assessment of patient with chest pain
  - Clinical examination skills

Professional leadership and consultancy

The most difficult part of the role for me was the leadership and consultancy element as I had what I thought to be little prior experience in this area. What made it even more difficult was that, from the outset, there was little clarity about who I would be leading or interacting with and at what level. While it was never a purpose of the NTC role to include managerial responsibilities, I found that the welcome omission of this responsibility meant there was a simultaneous, and not so welcome, loss of managerial authority. Therefore, initiatives or training could not be implemented in the fashion that I had been familiar with. Where previously I could organise the duty rota and let people know that I expected them to attend, I was now in the position of having to negotiate with the senior staff on duty to try to ensure a good attendance.

It is more straightforward to deal with medical staff in such a scenario as they have had a longstanding appreciation of the importance of ongoing learning and the need to take time out from the clinical area for this. Nurses, on the other hand, state that the excessive clinical workload takes precedence over education, and there is a reluctance to appreciate that a small investment of time in learning may actually pay dividends in terms of increased clinical awareness and improved quality of care. Busy clinical areas, combined with 12 hour shift working patterns, not only reduce the opportunity for, but also produce apathy towards, non-clinical activities. I tried to influence this negativity by targeting groups of student nurses who were supernumary to clinical needs. Delivering education that was positively appraised led to qualified nurses asking me questions about the sessions, initially on a one-to-one level but later in small groups. Achieving greater attendance at the teaching sessions was subsequently more successful when the initiative to arrange the sessions came from the qualified nurses themselves.

Extending nurse prescribing was an initiative that was proposed for our acute Trust soon after I took up post. Prior to the Crown II Report (DoH, 1999c), little consideration had been given to nurse prescribing in secondary care. Nurse prescribing had, however, been in the political arena since the late 1980s and had been successfully implemented in primary care for district nurses and health visitors (DoH, 1989). Exploring how extending the range of medications for prescription could be implemented in the acute Trust was deemed more than suitable for the Nurse Consultant role. Although I was initially sceptical about extended nurse prescribing owing to the limitations of the proposed new formulary, I soon realised that what was proposed could just be the tip of the iceberg and, if successfully implemented, might facilitate great improvements for patients.

After successfully completing the necessary training and a short period in practice, I accepted the lead position to try to develop the implementation further. Forming a local implementation group within the Trust has, first, helped to disseminate the latest developments for extended nurse prescribing. Second, it has also helped to run clinical supervision sessions for those nurses who have taken on a prescribing role in their practice or have taken it on as part of a new role. Third, this group addresses some of the continuing professional development needs.

With the little experience of prescribing that I felt I had, it is important to realise that being one of the first acute care-based nurses to develop with this remit has placed me at the forefront of experience, not only in my own practice, but also in terms of the information that I receive from the other nurses in our group. I therefore feel a great responsibility to share this experience with the army of individuals and disciplines who are also becoming involved in prescribing medication, either at an independent level or as supplementary practitioners. It was through discussions with others that I was, as mentioned earlier, invited to share my experiences.

I attend a vast array of committees and strategy groups as part of my role; some of these are listed in the summary of this key function. This was initially quite daunting as I frequently left some of the meetings wondering what language had been used and why everyone except me seemed to know what was being said. Occasionally hearing others say, 'What was that about?' was very comforting. As time has gone on, I have learned the 'language' and developed the confidence to offer my opinion when consulted or when I think it relevant. Now I come out of meetings thinking, 'Did I really say that?!'

Box 3.11   Summary of key function: professional leadership and consultancy

- Extended nurse prescribing
- CHD Workforce Development Confederation
- NSF CHD Local Implementation Team Clinical Sub-group
- Development of Tees-wide thrombolysis strategy
- Process review of RACPC referral between GPs and hospital
- Department of Health Nurse Consultants Groups
- Emergency care reforms

In summary, I hope that this case study will have provided you with an interesting example of the daily life and experiences of a current NTC, an understanding of the importance of the role in service development and an insight into how to establish yourself as a NTC.

RECOMMENDED READING

Dowling S (1996) Nurses taking on junior doctors' work: a confusion of accountability. *British Medical Journal* 312:1211–1214.

Leverson R, Vaughan B (1999) *Developing New Roles in Practice. An Evidence Based Guide*. Kings Fund/Sheffield University School of Policy Studies (SCHARR)/University of Bristol, London.

Manley K (2000) Organisational culture and nurse consultant outcomes. I. Organisational culture. *Nursing Standard* 14(36):34–38.

Manley K (2000) Organisational culture and nurse consultant outcomes. II. Nurse outcomes. *Nursing Standard* 14(37):34–38.

National Electronic Library for Health (NeLH), Virtual Branch, and Health Management.

Owen G (1998) Extended scope practitioners in orthopaedic outpatient clinics. *Rehabilitation International* Fall:33–34, 38.

Schön D.A. (1991) The Reflective Practitioner. Arena, Aldershot.

REFERENCES

Byrne P (2002) *Making the First Consultant Post Work*. Frontline CSP, London.

Department of Health (1989) *Report of the Advisory Group on Nurse Prescribing* (Crown Report). London, HMSO.

Department of Health (1999a) *Making a Difference: Strengthening the Nursing, Midwifery and Health Visiting Contribution to Health and Healthcare*. London,

Stationery Office.

Department of Health (1999b) *Nurse, Midwife and Health Visitor Consultants: Establishing Posts and Making Appointments*. Health Service Circular 217. HMSO, London.

Department of Health (1999c) *Review of Prescribing, Supply and Administration of Medicines Final Report* (Crown II Report). HMSO, London.

Department of Health (2000a) *Meeting the Challenge: A Strategy for the Allied Health Professions*. HMSO, London.

Department of Health (2000b) *The NHS Plan: A Plan for Investment, a Plan for Reform*. HMSO, London.

Department of Health (2000c) *National Service Framework for Coronary Heart Disease*. HMSO, London.

Department of Health (2001) Arrangement for consultant posts – staff covered by the professions allied to medicine. PT'A' Whitley Council Advance Letter AL PAM (PTA) 2/2001. DoH, Leeds.

Limb M (2003) *Opening new doors*. Frontline CSP, London.

Manley K (1997) A conceptual framework for advanced practice: an action research project operationalising an advanced practitioner/consultant nurse role. *Journal of Clinical Nursing* 6:179–190.

O'Dowd A (2000) Supernurses are go. *Nursing Times* 96(13):10–11.

4 GETTING STARTED AS A NURSE/THERAPIST CONSULTANT

Tim Renshaw

INTRODUCTION

The chapter builds on Chapter 3 by providing a framework for actioning the key themes and attributes associated with the Nurse/Therapist Consultant (NTC) post. The chapter focuses on providing practical advice and guidance on 'getting started' through my personal journey from being a specialist to a consultant nurse. Although some readers may think 'I am an allied health professional [AHP] or medical colleague, so why will this chapter be relevant to me?', please read on. This is because the advice, guidance, reflective questions and case studies may simply assist aspiring and existing NTCs in their roles in the future.

The chapter focuses on outlining important issues such as how to undertake an initial or baseline assessment linked to the job description, and key themes tied to the post. Furthermore, the importance of enhancing skills of self-awareness and critical reflection, along with the need for individual personal and professional development plans, is detailed. It is not my intention to try to provide answers to the many questions that are faced by newly appointed and experienced NTCs, asked of themselves and often by others.

When talking to peers, I discovered that my experiences were not unique: they are repeated and replayed in various forms nationally. Networking provides an opportunity to share and learn through these experiences. Once the euphoria of being appointed to such a post has subsided, a quiet reality will begin to dawn. In my case, my first question was, 'What have I taken on?', followed closely by 'Where do I begin?'

THE NTC: WHAT HAVE I TAKEN ON AND WHERE DO I BEGIN?

As outlined in Chapter 3, the roles and responsibilities of NTCs working in health and social care are vast, varied and complex. This may be because of the way in which each NTC post is designed to meet the specific requirements and characteristics of a unique organisational culture, management structure, set of clinical specialities and/or professional discipline. These unique characteristics associated with role, responsibilities and the context in which the NTC will work and operate are important to decipher. This is because they have the potential to influence the way in which the posts are operationalised and evaluated (Guest et al, 2001). Without doubt, the term 'Nurse/Therapist Consultant' seems to mean different things to different health care professionals and professional disciplines. This can be borne out by the ambiguity of its meaning in discussions with other NTCs and by reviewing the various job descriptions and early evaluation reports of NTCs over the past couple of years (Guest et al, 2001).

The initial challenge for any NTC in commencing these posts is where to start! At one end of the spectrum, you are excited; at the other end, you are apprehensive because of the fear of failure. But remember that these emotions and feelings are common to many NTCs, and indeed to most individuals who commence a new and pioneering position in health and social care.

All these factors and emotions make the NTC role unique because it is about individuals rising to the challenges imposed by the complexity and diversity of the role and responsibilities, different organisational cultures, clinical environments, workforce pressures, directional management/leadership and support. The NTC role provides hope and opportunity in health and social settings on several accounts because it is about:

- adopting a strategic position to facilitate and encourage modernisation
- making small/large changes in clinical, professional practice(s)
- encouraging developments in response to local, regional and national priorities and needs
- providing leadership and support to colleagues, peers and the public
- providing a career structure and pathway to aid recruitment and the retention of experienced and expert professionals in practice
- recognition of the health and social care professions for their contributions towards providing quality services within the context of a modernising National Health Service (NHS).

The challenge facing some NTCs in addressing all this lies in identifying, prioritising and balancing individual and organisational needs and demands. This is a highly important exercise and should not be neglected. Early occupiers of the NTC role will describe the importance of learning about the role and responsibility of the post by working through the challenges encountered as you endeavour to advance and evaluate the role and its responsibilities. According to the evaluation reports presented to date (Guest et al, 2001), the challenges facing the NTC are mainly associated with:

- raising staff and colleague awareness of the NTC
- clarifying the purpose, scope and remit of the NTC
- the NTC acquiring the knowledge skills, understanding, competence and confidence to establish and deliver the role and responsibilities
- taking the time and having the patience and persistence to understand that change needs time
- accepting that the NTC position is about accepting criticism, both positive and negative, providing that it is constructive and not destructive
- seeking help and support, and developing networks for sharing and disseminating information.

The challenges facing NTCs are in some ways similar to those facing colleagues who work in practice development because the role is concerned with facilitating *others* to innovate or evaluate practices through the establishment of partnerships, multiprofessional collaboration, effective communication and the sharing of the practice; in both cases, individuals fail to focus on their *own* personal/professional needs (McSherry, 2002).

Activity 4.1   *Reflective question*

Highlighting the diversity in the NTC's role and responsibilities

Having looked at your job description, note down what you see as the key roles and responsibilities associated with the post and how you plan to achieve them.

Read on and compare your findings with those in the Activity Feedback at the end of this section.

Activity 4.1 shows that it is important for NTCs to undertake this exercise in order to begin the process of developing, implementing and evaluating the position. There are many different and diverse self-assessment tools and techniques to assist you in this process, as highlighted in Table 4.1.

It is evident from Table 4.1 that several self-assessment tools and techniques are available from the business, marketing and health and social care organisations to help with prioritising and developing a strategy for 'getting started'. 'Self-assessment' in this case is about adopting and applying a suitable approach that will enable you to look at yourself and the organisation closely to see the systems the organisation has in place, in order to identify strengths and areas for further development. It is a structured tool asking NTCs, teams and the organisation to look at themselves against clearly defined measures, reflect on progress and think about future action. It also aids in planning and devising how to advance your role in the future.

When commencing my post, the Strengths, Weaknesses, Opportunities and Threats (SWOT) technique (McSherry and Pearce, 2002) proved to be a useful tool in the first months, helping in not only the development of the post, but also my personal development (Figure 4.1).

Strengths	Weaknesses
• Past knowledge	• Unknown to organisation
• Persistence	• Credibility
• Resilience	• Lack of clear role
• Expertise in field	• Strong sense of self
• Strong sense of self	• Leadership

Opportunities	Threats
• Unit meetings	• Isolation
• Working in wards	• Medical staff
• Find quick win	• Ambiguity
• Further training	• Not meeting others' expectations
• Links with local university	

Figure 4.1   SWOT analysis of an NTC post

Table 4.1   Initial assessment tools and techniques

Assessment tools and techniques	Brief definition	Potential use for the NTC	Use resource details
Political, Economical, Social and Technological Assessment (PEST analysis)	An organisation's operating environment can be analysed by looking at: • External forces (those factors over which an organisation has no control) • Internal forces (factors over which an organisation has direct control) The external environment of an organisation can be analysed by conducting a PEST analysis. This is a simple analysis of an organisation's political, economical, social and technological environment	Useful technique when exploring the long-term developments of the NTC position	Learning markets.net: http://www.learnmarketing. net/environment.htm
Strengths, Weaknesses, Opportunities and Threats (SWOT) analysis	SWOT analysis is commonly used in marketing as a tool to define plans and set strategies. 'SWOT' refers to the identification of strengths, weaknesses, opportunities and threats, and can help to define what needs to be done to adapt to new roles	Technique to be undertaken at the start of the role and periodically throughout. The use of development/action plans could be applied to support individual personal/professional development and the strategic development of the post	McSherry R, Pearce P (2002) Clinical Governance: A Guide to Implementation for Health Care Professionals. Blackwell Science Publications, Oxford MPS Healthcare: www.mps-ltd.com/ health care.pdf
Force Field Analysis (FFA)	A structured group analysis technique that attempts to maximise the success of a proposed solution. When you have agreed on a solution to a problem, you may well find the technique useful FFA is a way of identifying the forces and factors in place that support or work against your solution. You may then be able to develop some further ideas to reinforce the driving forces and reduce or eliminate the restraining forces	To establish and clarify the scope and purpose of the post Good technique for problem-solving	Force Field Analysis, University of Cambridge, Department of Engineering (2004) http://www.ifm.eng.cam.ac.uk/ dstools/represent/forcef.html./

| Impact Analysis (IA) | IA is a tool that can be used to help. (It is worth spending an appropriate amount of time making sure that you have defined the problem properly before you set out on an improvement project. No matter how clever we are at coming up with solutions to problems, if we are working on the wrong problems in the first place we are wasting our time.) It is an excellent way for a team of people to start thinking about a problem, and it often serves as an early pointer to possible solutions. Like all the tools and techniques, it is easy to do but can make a big difference (NHS, 2004) | An excellent technique to use for seeking views and opinions in the early stages 'for getting started' in the role | The National Health Service (2004) The Improvement Network: Connecting People with Knowledge and Innovation http://www.tin.nhs.uk/sys_upl/templates/StdLeft/StdLeft_disp.asp?pgid=1376&tid=144 |
| Corporate, management and clinical self-assessment tools | The assessment tools provided by the Commission for Health Inspection and Audit (CHIa) provide useful tools and templates for establishing the overall systems, processes, standards and quality at an individual, team and organistional level | These self-assessment tools and could be modified and used to assist you in establishing the initial or baseline assessment | Healthcare Commission http://www.health care commission.org.uk/Information ForServiceProviders/Selfassessment. |

Figure 4.1 shows that it was possible, from the SWOT analysis, to draw a development and strategic plan, which over the next months changed and developed as my personal experience and organisational awareness developed. Essentially, the SWOT analysis became a key tool in my survival kit. This allowed me to identify the breadth of the role and, more importantly, the skills required to achieve the goals identified in the role description. From the combination of these two simple yet essential techniques, a number of deficiencies were identified regarding my level of training that needed to be addressed to enable me to act more effectively in the NTC role, for example undertaking prescribing and clinical examination skills. The SWOT analysis is an ideal assessment to help you deal with the early emotions and experiences that you will encounter.

EARLY EMOTIONS AND EXPERIENCES

When the day finally arrives and you accept the post, you are beginning a journey unlike any other you have started in your career. In my case, I had spent nearly 25 years working in the same organisation, developing trusting relationships with colleagues. Now I was moving into a new role in a new organisation, leaving my past behind and moving into a new future. The feelings and emotions can be summarised into four themes: emotional roller-coaster, meeting and greeting, role ambiguity, and engaging the patient and public through seeking an expectation of services.

Emotional roller-coaster

Excitement and trepidation were the key emotions in my early days in post, and it is good to see that my experience was shared with other NTCs (Guest et al, 2001). What seemed to help to resolve these emotions, and make 'getting started' a little easier, was having an orientation programme in the first month to help with the initial settling-in process.

It was interesting to see that there was, within the senior level of management, one preconceived notion of what the NTC post would achieve, whereas at grass-roots level there was another (not necessarily matching) idea. Indeed, some clinical colleagues held the belief that the NTCs should work on their clinical areas almost as an extra pair of hands when staffing was short. An important early lesson was the need for communication about the role itself so staff got to know me and, more importantly, what the post would do for them. This was coupled with an interesting experience during induction in which all the attendees stood up and introduced themselves; I spent a good 20 minutes with the group, discussing the role and its implications. The interest shown in the NTC post was excellent, making the meeting and greeting of staff, patients and public a top priority.

The importance of meeting and greeting

The importance of meeting and greeting gave me my first and important objective, the need to 'meet the people and discuss the post'. At the *Nursing*

Standard Nurse of the Year Award Ceremony in 1998, the Prime Minister, Tony Blair, announced plans to create 'Supernurses' (latterly therapists) who would ideally share the same status as medical consultants (Harker, 2001). The aim of this role was to offer an alternative career path for experienced nurses that would allow them to remain in direct patient contact and 'provide an opportunity to implement a patient-centred model of care' (Jones, 2002). The debates that followed the launch of these posts and the potential for modernisation continue to this day. A recurring issue for taking forward the role and responsibilities of the NTC seems to be associated with role ambiguity and with defining the scope and remit of the post.

Role ambiguity

Role ambiguity seems to be emerging because NTCs, professionals, patients and the public are unclear what the posts mean and involve for them. Similarly, they are receiving mixed messages through the media, making it difficult for them to see the potential and opportunity that these posts hold for modernisation in the NHS (Jones, 2002).

The Royal College of Nursing (BBC News online network 1998) stated that 'although it welcomed the announcement of the Nurse Consultant there were already supernurses or expert nurses in post but who were not paid for their extended roles'. With the growing number and diversity of titles within nursing, and indeed the allied health professions (Figure 4.2), there is always a concern that patients and their carers will be uncertain who they are actually seeing. An editorial from the *Journal of Clinical Medicine* (2002) raised the fact that, with the

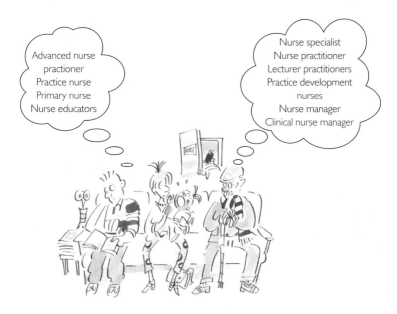

Figure 4.2   Examples of nurse titles

development of new nursing (in parallel AHP) roles, there has been a reduction in the number of experienced nurses in general nursing areas, which has in turn led to a decline in standards in hospital wards in the United Kingdom. This may be an oversimplification of a very complex manpower issue that is currently affecting all disciplines within the health and social care arena – some professions more than others (DoH, 1999).

Hopefully, Figure 4.2 is not a full or even a partial representation of patients, the public image, experiences of nursing and indeed AHP services. It is fundamentally important that the role of the NTC is not stereotyped into an image before it has had time to become an essential position within nursing and the AHP disciplines. To avoid this, it is important that patients' and the public's expectations and experiences are sought, listened to and acted upon.

Engaging the patient and public through seeking an expectation of services

The Wanless Report (2002) identified that a key driver for health and social care over the next 20 years was patients' expectations of services. The report indicated that patients would in future expect fast access to integrated patient-centred services in a safe environment with comfortable accommodation, which focused on ensuring quality. There would be a move from informed consent to informed choice, with acute hospitals concentrating upon specialist care (Wanless, 2002). A major issue is currently capacity, and the key to addressing this is the workforce. The development of new ways of working and new roles will contribute to addressing this issue. It is precisely here that the NTC might be able to have a major impact through the development of alternative methods of health and social care provision and the empowerment of colleagues to ensure that this approach continues. The implementation of key roles such as that of the NTC requires clear forethought and planning.

Activity 4.1　Feedback _____

Highlighting the diversity in the NTC's role and responsibilities

The NTC's role and responsibilities are complex, diverse and unique to each individual position. This is because each organisation has its own systems, structures, culture, working environment and management and leadership styles/approaches in place that are not replicable elsewhere in the NHS. Encouraging NTCs to 'get started' requires a detailed self-assessment to be undertaken and a personal/professional and strategic development plan(s) to be developed so that NTCs can move forward in advancing and evaluating modernisation. The job description and business case may provide some practical advice and guidance to aid this process. It is, however, worth mentioning that the latter will be challenging in the light of possible role ambiguities and will require a firm commitment to meeting and greeting colleagues, the public and patients, along with listening and responding to their expectations.

PREPARING YOURSELF TO UNDERTAKE THE ROLE OF AN NTC

Preparing yourself to undertake the role of an NTC is difficult, challenging yet overwhelmingly exciting. The key to successful preparation is not to leave it too late. It could, for example, be argued that your preparation begins when you first obtain the job description, specification and application forms.

Activity 4.2   *Reflective question*

Preparing to undertake the role of an NTC

Write down what you think is necessary when preparing to undertake the NTC role.

Read on and compare your findings with those in the Activity Feedback at the end of this section.

It is evident from Activity 4.2 that preparation for undertaking the role and responsibilities of the NTC could be based on adopting a phased approach, as outlined in Table 4.2.

Table 4.2   Phase approach to preparing and undertaking the role of the NTC

Phase	Approaches	Rationale
Pre-interview selection	*Reviewing* the job description and specification *Clarifying* the reasons, scope and purpose of the post *Ensuring* that you have the qualifications, knowledge, skills and competence to undertake the role and responsibilities *Preparing* to undertake the selection process: 'fact-finding' by visiting, communicating and sharing your ideas with potential employers and staff to identify similarities	A review of the job description for the post will begin to tell you the purpose, scope and remit of the post and its requirements, as well as the type of person that the organisation is looking for
Post-selection – appointment	*Preparing and planning* a strategy for success by: *Exploring* ways of undertaking self-assessments, and the initial assessment *Researching and reviewing* your ideas and visions for the post	To formulate what you consider to be the structure of the role that addresses the organisational need for the post
Commencing the post	*Informing and engaging* your vision through seeking views and opinions *Communicating*, networking and sharing your vision and plans *Developing* a series of objectives and a implementation and action plan *Undertaking* an initial assessment so that progress can be monitored and evaluated *Devising* a process of *implementation* for a pattern of role engagement	To establish a robust system(s) and frameworks for implementing and evaluating the post

Table 4.2   *continued*

Twelve-monthly review	*Reviewing* and *evaluating* progress to date	This is fundamental to establishing how the post is developing and to seeing whether objectives, timescales, the personal development and implementation action plan, etc. are realistic and representative of the post-holder. To clarify the role and responsibilities of the post and to share strengths and areas for further development
Evaluation	An essential phase that should be incorporated throughout all the phases. As an NTC you should liaise with research and development, audit departments and any other organisational departments that could support you in devising a structured approach to evaluating the NTC position. When preparing and undertaking the role, the evaluation could be based on the phase to preparing and evaluating the role	High-priority aspect of the role in demonstrating the overall efficiency and effectiveness of the post and impacts on individual, public/patient, organisational and regional/national levels

NB: The above is only a guide and is not intended to be prescriptive or to show any order of priority when preparing and undertaking the role of the NTC. Furthermore, it is not an exhaustive list of ideas and ways for preparing, implementing and evaluating the role.

According to a critical review and synthesis of the evaluative literature presented by Watson (2002), Guest et al (2001) and Ward et al (1998), successful preparation seems to be based on adopting a phased and sequential approach to advancing and evaluating the role. According to Table 4.2, the phased approach can be based on five phases: pre-interview selection, post-selection – appointment, commencing the post, 12-monthly review and planning for evaluation. This phased approach to preparing and undertaking the NTC role is essential to ensure that the post-holder has sufficient time to settle in and 'take up' the post. Furthermore, the NTC requires plenty of time to acquire ideas and share and disseminate information so that both the NTC and other staff familiarise themselves with the scope, purpose, breadth and remit of the post.

In brief, *phase 1* would be reviewing the job description for the post, which begins to identify the purpose, scope and remit of the post and its requirements, as well as the type of person that the organisation is looking for. As outlined in Chapter 3, each post that is advertised will have a theme that may be linked to the government agenda for health care. Whether that relates to the older person or emergency care, the primary driver will be easily identifiable and researchable.

Phase 2 – preparation for the interview process – leads you to formulate what you consider to be the structure of the role that addresses the organisational need for the post, the governmental aspirations for the post, the professional concept of what the post means and, most importantly, your own personalised image of how the post could function and how you would begin to structure the post.

Once appointed to the post, you 'take up' the role. *Phase 3* is essential for starting to clarify your aspirations and initial ideas of how these match perceptions of the role by staff, colleagues, patients and the public. Strategies for introducing the post should be formulated and the necessary steps taken to undertake an initial baseline and self-assessment. This permits an overall picture of how the post may begin to emerge so that development plans can be written and realistic time-frames established.

Phase 4, the 12-monthly review, could be undertaken to establish the strengths and areas for improvement of the post. The review should focus on establishing whether the aims, objectives and development plans following the initial baseline and self-assessments were realistic and achievable. This review relates to learning from current experiences and encounters so that firm preparations and planning can be made to inform the long-term evaluation of the post.

Phase 5, it may be argued, is the most fundamental aspect of preparing for the NTC role in order to ensure long-term survival. This is because the phase concerns demonstrating the efficiency and effectiveness of the role. Evaluation needs to be directed and focused on several levels, for example:

Individual
• NTC
• staff
• patient(s)
Organisational
• improving access
• achieving targets
• enhancing career structures
• recruitment and retention
• value for money.

Evaluation is covered in more detail in Chapter 8. A phased approach to undertaking the NTC post ensures that role engagement can be affirmed and the necessary plans made to begin the processes of operationalising and evaluating the post. Preparing for and undertaking the NTC role will not occur without the necessary support of the organisation, managers and professional colleagues.

Preparation: the importance of organisational, managerial and peer support

Developing Key Roles for Nurses and Midwives: A Guide for Managers (DoH, 2002) produced some practical advice and guidance for managers that can be used to support NTCs in preparing for and undertaking their role (see Table 4.3 below). In practice, many of the tips apply to the nurse or AHP who is embarking on an NTC post. It is evident from Activity 4.2 that the role of the NTC is exciting, challenging yet fraught with potential difficulties because these are new posts with no underlying history or foundations. The first occupiers are essentially the pioneers laying the foundation for others to build on. There is, however, no doubt that NTCs will feel as if they are under the spotlight.

So what can managers, employers and NTCs do to get things off to a good start? The DoH (2002) has provided some initial practical advice and guidance, which the author has adapted in the light of his experiences and reflections as an

NTC (Table 4.3). Although the advice and guidance in the table is sound, it reinforces previous arguments that NTCs need to be selective in prioritising their workload so that the patterns of engagement in the role are supportive and representative of the purpose, scope and remit of the post.

Table 4.3   Developing key roles: tips for managers and NTCs

	Top tips for managers	**Practitioner comments**
Getting started	• Be clear about the aims • Define the objectives • Look at practice change • Identify benefits for the organisation • Start small • Don't try to do it all at once • Develop protocols • Don't reinvent the wheel	• Have a vision • Focus • Limit what you can do • Don't be all things to all people
Supporting staff	• Train your staff and allow time • Prepare your staff educationally • Key roles need support and development • Remember the stresses on staff • Establish clinical supervision • Develop your staff • Staff are the key to change	• Set realistic goals • It takes time to change • Supervision is essential • Training is crucial
Ensuring ownership	• Project lead • Let staff develop the changes • Change from the bottom up • Allow the use of the word 'no' • Satisfied staff stay	• Allow the freedom to say 'no', particularly when you are exceeding your expertise
Communication	• Don't let staff get isolated • Meet colleagues to exchange ideas • Get support from colleagues • Publicise changes • Be flexible • Have a sense of humour • Inform staff of the benefits of change	• Keep clinicians' support • Remember the 'feel-good factor' • Keep the service profile high
Structure and funding	• Adequate clerical support • Identify mainstream funding	• Be creative in securing funding
Audit and evaluation	• Audit against credible standards • If it doesn't work, be honest • Don't give up	• Audit is key and needs to be built in at an early stage

Adapted from Department of Health (2002).

Role and patterns of engagement

As mentioned in previous chapters, the NTC's role is built around four key dimensions: expert practice, education and training, research, and leadership. On paper, each of these functions is of equal importance to the role, but individual NTCs will attach differing importance to these depending on their personal experience and preference, and in order to accommodate the needs of the post.

A common expectation within these posts, one that is frequently made explicit, is the notion that NTCs will spend 50% of their time in the clinical field and 50%

of their time addressing the four key functions. At face value, this appears to be a rational division of workload, but in practice it can cause personal and role conflicts and role/workload overload for new post-holders. How, for example, do you undertake and deliver all four dimensions of the role when you do not know what is a priority? Similarly, is it possible to have a clinical caseload and sufficient time to contribute to developing new ideas for research?

Where posts are of a traditional format, tried and tested, a new post-holder will have a good idea what to expect and, once in post, has a historical foundation from which to work. NTC posts are still in their infancy, and their effectiveness is still under evaluation, so new post-holders will find themselves in a role that has no clear definition and is laced with ambiguity. There is the feeling of being the leaders and pioneers of the profession, leading the nursing and the allied health professions 'to boldly go' into the new world. Herein may lie the ultimate appeal of the role. While the role remains ambiguous, there is the opportunity to stamp your own personality upon it, to develop it in the way that you feel best achieves the goals of the job description. However, the true value of these posts is found not in the individual but in the sustainability and durability of the post. For here is the true test and challenge of these posts: when post-holders move on, is there a need to replace them and to continue to develop the role, or is the post left unfilled, those activities being taken on and absorbed by others?

Manley (1997) identifies six core skills and qualities that are required by a Consultant Nurse (Therapist) to ensure that the NTC survives in the future:

1 Be able to apply the practice of nursing [therapy] to a specific client group, whether as a generalist or a specialist.
2 Have leadership and strategic vision.
3 Be able to use research and evaluation approaches that focus on day-to-day issues in everyday practice.
4 Facilitate practice development and structural, cultural and practice change.
5 Create a learning culture, one that enables all members of the interdisciplinary team to learn and develop their potential.
6 Provide consultancy – from a clinical level in relation to individual patients to an organisational level in terms of the provision of patient-centred services.

If NTCs can ensure that their role and patterns of engagements contribute to the successful achievement of Manley's core qualities, replacing NTCs and ensuring successors to existing NTC positions will undeniably follow. As many NTCs currently 'fear failure', the difficulty for some NTCs will be ensuring that they establish sufficient credibility to deliver the role successfully.

Credibility: its importance to the NTC

The second early objective identified was achieving credibility, defined by Chambers (2004) as 'one being reliable and trustworthy in order that they are believed'. It soon became evident that, to have some level of acceptance and credibility, NTCs needed to adopt a simple strategy. My choice was to combine observing the clinical areas with working on these areas, adopting set shifts including nights. This provided an opportunity to get to know the staff and to see at first hand how the systems worked.

To support the development of my strategy, it was useful to enhance my credibility by attending a number of seminars and meetings held by nursing, medical and management staff to discuss the role and my vision. As with any new role, there are supporters, those 'on the fence' and opposition; interestingly, it can be difficult to predict where one's supporters and opponents will come from – it is always advisable to expect the unexpected. Some of the most interesting and trying discussions involved my medical and nursing colleagues, as illustrated in Box 4.1.

Box 4.1   Personal reflection: highlighting the importance of credibility

At a senior medical meeting that involved both acute and secondary care staff, I was asked to present the Nurse Consultant role. It became clear that the majority were apathetic to what I had told them, some had a problem with the title 'Consultant' as this was traditionally a medical title, and others wanted to know what duties I would be taking away from the junior medical staff.

On reflection, I believe that the key to this discussion was the emphasis on demonstrating my credibility through the nursing aspect of the role and the development of nursing. I do not believe that a Nurse Consultant should be expected to pick up those roles which medical staff deem fit to drop. Taking on roles from other professional groups needs to be carefully considered, asking the question 'Do I need to do this?'

What emerges from the reflection in Box 4.1 is that other nursing and AHP colleagues hold a variety of perceptions surrounding the NTC. Some cannot grasp the difference between an NTC and a Nurse/Therapist Specialist and Practitioner, a point eloquently deciphered by Jones (2002). They feel cheated if an NTC is not in their clinical area every day and does not grasp the complexity of the role. To address these issues of identity and credibility, it was important to develop a strategy or strategies circumventing the problems. 'I do not feel that I am being unfair when I say that as professionals we can be very self-critical particularly when there is a new post and role developed' (Jones, 2002).

Activity 4.2   Feedback

Preparing to undertake the role of an NTC

In brief, preparing to undertake the role of the NTC is difficult, challenging and rewarding. A possible way forward to ensure successful preparation for and undertaking of the NTC role is to adopt a phased approach to development, implementation and evaluation, focusing on the potential aspects of the role that may create conflict, for example by defining the role and patterns of engagement and credibility.

The remainder of this chapter presents two case studies to assist and support aspiring and existing NTCs with 'getting started'. The way forward is to share and learn with and from each other, and to be constructively critical rather than hypercritical. These are personal case studies to show my personal strategy and what worked for me.

CONCLUSION

Finally, I recently sat with a group of NTCs listening to a fascinating discussion about titles – whether the title Nurse/Therapist Consultant or Consultant Nurse/Therapist should be used, and when does one become the other? My advice is never to forget your professional origin. I am a nurse who has been given the opportunity through this post to make a real contribution to the profession of nursing, to health care and, most importantly, to our patients and their carers. They are, after all, our reason for being.

SUMMARY OF KEY POINTS

- Early occupiers of the NTC role will tell you of the importance of learning about the role and responsibility of the post by working through the challenges encountered as you endeavour to advance and evaluate the role and its responsibility(s).
- There are many different and diverse self-assessment tools and techniques to assist you in preparing for and undertaking the role.
- 'Getting started' requires a detailed self-assessment to be undertaken and a personal/professional and strategic development plan(s) to be prepared in order to move forward in advancing and evaluating modernisation.
- The job description and business case may provide some practical advice and guidance to help with undertaking a self-assessment exercise and writing the strategy and action plan.
- Preparation for undertaking the role and responsibilities of the NTC could be based on adopting a phased approach to development, implementation and evaluation.
- NTC roles are at the cutting edge of health and social care in encouraging changes in practice in modern times. With the autonomy attached to these roles, the NTC may not be an easy transition to adapt to, but it is definitely exciting and rewarding.
- For more practical advice and guidance for 'getting started', refer to the checklist in Box 4.2.

Box 4.2 Getting started as an NTC: a practical advice and guidance checklist

Tick when completed/experienced

- Read around the post and develop an understanding of what the role brings to health care.
- Meet with a current post-holder and if possible spend some time working with him or her.
- Find out what the organisation expects from the post-holder.
- Identify what support services are available or will be made available as the post develops.
- Identify any training or development needs you have and actively pursue them.
- Expect ambiguity.
- Realise that there will be good and bad days.
- Expect to be frustrated.
- Build and keep your links with the senior management of your organisation.
- Do not expect to be welcomed by everyone you meet.
- Keep your allies close to you; keep your opponents closer.
- Expect to be criticised.
- Expect to have to work hard.
- Develop your clinical workload as soon as possible.
- Plan to keep control of your workload.
- Focus on your objectives: do not be distracted or waylaid.
- Find a good mentor as soon as possible.
- Network locally and nationally.
- Tie into Department of Health-led groups if possible, or contact the Department of Health to help you identify any leads who can be of help to you.
- Develop a clinical supervision group locally with other consultants.
- If you do not currently have the skill, develop the ability to say 'no'.
- Be realistic with your own expectation of what one person can achieve in post.
- Be prepared to describe the post to colleagues.
- Do not apologise for your post.
- Be seen to be consistent at work.
- Listen to others.
- Communicate your intentions.
- Acknowledge failures.
- Do not panic if you are not fulfilling all four key functions: remember your workload.
- Whenever possible, further develop your leadership skills.
- Keep a high profile both internally and externally to the organisation.
- Give yourself time in the week to think and plan.
- Do not forget to go home occasionally – your partner will appreciate it!

CASE STUDY 4.1 MARKETING: ITS IMPORTANCE IN RAISING AWARENESS AND THE PROFILE OF THE **NTC**

Tim Renshaw

Raising colleagues' awareness of NTC post(s) is essential to achieving 'early-win' situations. The challenges and difficulties when commencing a new post relate, however, to how to achieve early wins! A possible way forward is to share and disseminate information pertaining to the purpose, scope and remit of the post, along with its key role and responsibilities within the organisation.

Figure 4.3 outlines some practical advice and guidance for getting started in the post, this being discussed in the remaining sections.

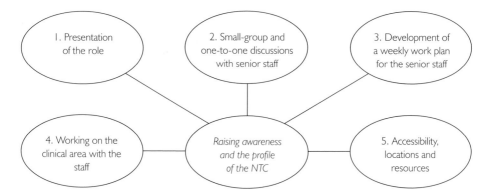

Figure 4.3   Getting started: some practical advice and guidance for raising awareness and the profile of the NTC

1.   Presentation of the role

This approach was used at both directorate and unit meetings. Each venue required a slightly different emphasis for the presentation. Although never openly asked, the underlying questions revolved around:

- What do we get from this post?
- What are you going to do for us?
- What form will your work take on my ward?

The key message for nursing staff is to emphasise the benefits for the identified patient groups and to work with the clinically based staff to help them to develop their services. The key message for the medical staff was that this post was to function as a partnership but that it was a nursing post rather than a post on which they could dump the duties that they would prefer to avoid.

2.   Small-group and one-to-one discussions with senior staff

This forum was used to further deliver the message of the Nurse Consultant role and help to identify possible areas of development. The small-group approach encouraged an informal and safe environment for discussing issues.

3.   Development of a weekly work plan for the senior staff

The main concern of the staff, and the area of least understanding, was what the role entailed. Once the post had become established, the weekly work plan helped the staff to understand the workload of the Nurse Consultant post and grasp the breadth of the role. The problem with this approach was that, as the role developed, the work plan also evolved and changed, although it served its purpose.

4.   Working on the clinical area with the staff

Although this can also be of some use, you need to be careful and clear in relation to the aim of working in this way. If your aim is to identify developmental issues with the clinical teams, this is valid. If, however, you are there to make up numbers in the face of a crisis, then, although this is invaluable from a 'credibility' viewpoint, the actual potential for benefit can be limited, the knock-on effect being that you use up some of your limited and valuable time, which you can ill-afford to waste.

There is no right or wrong here: you will need to understand what is happening in the clinical areas, and it is helpful if clinical staff understand your role. In personal terms, the greatest benefit is to be gained from small-group meetings and working on clinical areas. By choosing when and where to work, you can control time usage and, as an outsider coming into the organisation, create the opportunity to see at grass-roots level how the clinical areas work.

5.   Accessibility, locations and resources

It is important to be accessible, easily located and sufficiently resourced to perform the role and responsibilities of the NTC to a high standard. Accessibility and location go hand in hand because colleagues need to be able to see you, speak to you and, more importantly, access your knowledge, skills, expertise and experience. Location is therefore an important factor to consider in getting started and settled in the NTC position: do you have an office near to your speciality or somewhere else in the organisation? This decision should not be made lightly but in consultation and collaboration with your colleagues, users and existing NTC post-holders. Key to any new role are the resources put into it, and although it is fair to say that resource requirements are minimal in the early, formative days, there are basic essential needs (Box 4.3).

Box 4.3   Resource requirements to meet the needs of the NTC

- Office: a base and space to work in and from
- IT links
- Laptop
- Stationery budget
- Training budget
- Mobile phone
- Travel budget
- Pager

It is almost incomprehensible to think that the basic resources outlined in Box 4.3 would not be made available to any newly appointed NTC. At the interview, however, or before accepting the post, it is worth checking what resources will be available to the successful applicant. Not clarifying this information may mean that, from your first day in post, you are not provided with enough resources. Do not assume that practical issues associated with resources are or have been organised. I would argue that these resources are the least that should be in place on day one, enabling new post-holders to start the planning phase of the role and giving the impression of positive planning by and support from the organisation. Alas, this is not always the case. My conversations with other NTCs nationally record great variation: one NTC had nothing and had to work from the car, keeping the notes in the car boot during the day. This is clearly unacceptable and fortunately an exception rather than the rule.

But what about the question of administrative or secretarial support? In some network meetings, a few NTCs are almost obsessional about administrative/secretarial support, which appears to be an issue of 'status'. I would argue that, until the post is established and you know your boundaries and the parameters of the post, you should hold back from seeking administrative/secretarial support. Although administrative/secretarial support may create a 'feel-good factor', it may initially be unnecessary and indeed boring for the support person, who could have little to do in the early stages of post development. Conversely, administrative/secretarial support in the early stages might help the NTC and the wider team to adapt and evolve into the role together.

In summary, it is important for NTCs to develop a strategy in the early stages of their post that is directed towards raising awareness and profiling the purpose, scope, role and responsibilities of the position. For this, both marketing and resourcing are essential. Having identified the importance of marketing and profiling the NTC post, the challenge may then lie in undertaking a 'baseline' or 'initial' assessment so that markers can be set, monitored and evaluated in order to demonstrate the long-term outcomes of the post.

Tim Renshaw

The realisation of beginning: 'a good beginning makes a good ending'

To demonstrate the efficiency and effectiveness – or 'outcome(s)' – of the NTC, it is essential to establish a baseline or initial assessment of existing service provision, standards and quality of services and organisational structures, cultures and working environment. This is important to show how the NTC post evolves and to provide a framework for implementing, monitoring and evaluating it.

The initial self-assessment, as already highlighted, involved undertaking a SWOT analysis as well as a review of government reforms and policy documents, a critical review and a role analysis of the job description, raising my awareness of political agendas and establishing a pattern of engagement. This case study outlines my reflections since occupying the post.

Review of government reforms and policy documents

Once you have had time to settle into the post and the induction programme has run its course, it is necessary to return to the job description to study in depth and critically extract what is expected of you. In some cases, this is reasonably straightforward; in others, things may not be as clear. This lack of clarity often arises from general uncertainties surrounding what the post actually concerns. In the current ever-changing climate of health and social care, the political drive is for a better utilisation of services, better access and better patient choice. Supporting these political agendas are a number of policy documents, for example the *National Service Framework* (NSF) *for Older People* (DoH, 2001), which has been produced to target and develop services for the older person. Most NTC posts have NSFs to support their work, and it is from these that Trusts have to develop strategies and derive targets to achieve. It therefore makes sense to use these policy documents as a focus for work.

Critical review and role analysis of the job description

The job description, although ambiguous and sometimes confusing, will be your primary tool to identify your starting position when in post. As stated in the Department of Health (2002) guide for managers on developing key roles, you cannot take everything on at once. Trying this and failing will lead to personal dissatisfaction and harm the credibility of the post. Never underestimate others' expectations of this post and what it will do for them. Use the time spent meeting your clinical and nursing leads to decide an action plan based on your observations of the organisation, the job description and where you feel that you can make an impact in the short term. In tandem with this, also decide a long-term objective that will make a larger impact, allowing more time for its development.

Political agendas

Regardless of our political stance, it is essential to be politically aware in post. None of us is exempt from or immune to the political environments in which we work. By being aware of this, NTCs will be able to work in a number of challenging forums and hopefully be more successful. This aspect is sometimes referred to as being aware of the 'big p's' and 'little p's'.

The 'big p's' refer to the national political agenda – not just the policy documents and advisory notices that come down from central government, but also the issues underlying these government statements. It is very important to tie into this important area as soon as possible. Some may find this a daunting prospect, wondering where to begin. You are unlikely to receive an invitation to London to talk strategy so you will need to find a way in. The Department of Health website provides access to a number of network groups, whose lead individuals you can contact. This will be a key access point to influence strategy nationally and, with work, will open up other avenues. Although time-consuming, it can prove to be very worthwhile, particularly as you develop your role and work towards changing national practice. It can also provide a mine of useful information to influence your future decisions.

The 'little p's' are the politics that you will encounter within your working environment and organisation. We all have our own personal politics, agendas and motivations, in roles that are clearly laid out with a specific format and little true autonomy: the ward sister's sphere of influence is, for example, limited to perhaps just one clinical area. When working, it is, regardless of the situation, very useful to understand the function of the situation and also appreciate others' concerns and agendas. It is easier to work with the people than against them, particularly if they hold the key to a project's success. As an NTC, you are in a curious position not often experienced within nursing and perhaps the allied health professions: you will find yourself with influence and power across a range of clinical and non-clinical areas.

After I had undertaken these strategies, it was possible through personal interpretation to decipher government and organisational priorities. This was essential in the initial development and in establishing a pattern of engagement for the post.

Establishing a pattern of engagement

The next step was to look at how the role would function in relation to the four key themes and the strategic component of the role. As previously stated, the post is often split up into 50% clinical work and 50% 'other' work related to the post. When considering the role, it is necessary to take into account the four key functions, and I will consider here each of these functions in relation to my own personal experience.

Leadership

Health Service Circular 1999/217 (DoH, 1999b) states that:

> consultant practitioners will be appointed to senior practice based posts comprising a significant professional function. Posts will need to be structured to create the conditions that support and enable jobholders to exercise leadership to support and inspire colleagues, to improve standards and quality and to develop professional practice.

Leadership skills and qualities are a fundamental requirement of Nurse Consultant posts. Without such skills, I would argue that the post-holder is probably in the wrong job, but I concede that this is not a major issue at this level. We all have varying levels of leadership skills, and many Nurse Consultants have attended a range of leadership training and development days as part of their ongoing personal development. There is, however, a difference here that needs to be remembered: as Nurse Consultants, we have a responsibility to lead nursing into the future, and this applies equally to our therapy consultants. It is not just about a new grade of nursing, a new career path. We have a duty towards our professions and the general public to develop the services that are provided to meet public expectations. We have been given an opportunity to make significant changes in health care. Central to this, and a major determinant of success, are the leadership skills of the individual post-holder.

I realised this quite early in the post, and with this came concerns that my leadership skills were not as comprehensive as I felt they needed to be. Here I was fortunate in having the full support of my organisation. From my SWOT analysis, I had identified that my current MSc course was probably not the best one to be undertaking, particularly as it was heavily based in the sciences, biomechanics and maths. My first decision was to discontinue this course and start a new Master's degree that included leadership components. I was also fortunate at that time to be part of a network of Nurse Consultants for older people who, in meetings with representatives from the Department of Health, had identified the importance of leadership in these roles and the need for further personal development in this area. In conjunction with the NHS Leadership Centre, we have all been given access to a leadership development programme that has proved to be highly useful.

Expert practice

NTCs will be expected to provide expert advice across a multitude of professions at both local and strategic levels internally and externally to the organisation employing them, as reported in Health Service Circular 1999/217 (DoH, 1999b). Benner (1984) states that:

> expertise in complex human decision making, such as nursing requires, makes the interpretation of clinical situations possible, and the knowledge embedded in this clinical expertise is central to the advancement of nursing practice and the development of nursing science.

Therefore the expert NTC can notice those subtle physiological changes in a patient's condition and take the necessary steps. Those who label this as intuition or gut feeling will not have the depth of knowledge or experience to identify these physiological changes and the underlying pathophysiology involved.

When I started this post, I considered myself to be an expert in trauma and orthopaedics as it had been my specialism for 20 years and I carried the appropriate qualifications and depth of experience. The focus of the post I had taken up was the older person and rehabilitation following fractures. The mechanics of trauma caused me no problem, but treating the older person is often complex. As we all know, the majority of older people who are in hospital with a fracture usually have problems arising from multiple pathologies, the fracture being the least of their problems. My concern was that I had some limitations in relation to the pathology of ageing and the associated conditions; if I was the expert, I would need to address this deficit. I adopted a combination strategy consisting of:

- finding a physician who would be prepared to allow me on the teaching rounds
- the completion of a clinical examination skills course at the local university.

This increased my study workload in the first year but was necessary for both the post and my personal self-confidence. It would, however, have been easier not to have followed this course, but as an autonomous practitioner running my own clinics, managing my own caseload and following up patients with a fracture of the femoral neck, I felt that the patient had to be treated as a whole person – it was therefore essential to identify other problems associated with age. If experts in a small field become too specialised, they cannot and do not fully benefit their patients. The risk is, as Nicholas Murray Butler (1862–1947) stated, that 'an expert is one who knows more and more about less and less'. I advise any NTC to consider this. Because of this danger of overspecialisation, identify what your role relates to, who your client group is and what knowledge will you need to best benefit your clients. You cannot be an expert in everything, but consider what you are trying to achieve and what is expected of you.

Education

In conjunction with expert practice, there is a requirement that the post-holder will become actively involved in developing the education of health care staff. There will probably be a focus on experienced colleagues who are developing advanced skills; they in turn will cascade this knowledge down to their teams (DoH, 1999b).

The educational aspect of the posts will again focus on the needs of the post. This can be broadly divided into two sections: internal and external to the organisation. Within the organisation, you may, as the expert in a particular field, receive requests to attend various seminars to present information on a variety of issues. It is advisable to familiarise yourself with the organisation, identify your specific objectives in relation to the role and identify any training that is currently ongoing or any areas in which there is a need for training and education.

External to the organisation, there is an expectation on the part of the local university, who probably had a representative on the interview panel, that you will spend time in their institution working on various modules at pre- and postregistration levels. You could be offered an Honorary Lecturership to cement this relationship further.

Research

As a Consultant, part of the role, which links with the other key functions, is research. The development of evidence-based practice and the implementation of this evidence base are core to the role. This does not necessarily mean, however, that the NTC has personally to lead research; instead, the role is more one of supporting and assisting other practitioners in their research pursuits. It is, however, essential that the NTC at some point leads a specific piece of research that will contribute to the body of knowledge and, more importantly, give the post-holder credibility as a researcher.

All this demonstrates the complexity and difficulties that an NTC may experience in engaging and delivering the role. Having performed the role for several years and had the time to reflect upon the past, what I have learnt may make things a little easier for existing, new and aspiring NTCs.

Reflecting on the past: a personal overview

When you are successful in being offered an NTC post, there is often a great excitement and sense of a new challenge, a time of change. Although I had studied the job description at length before starting in post, the reality of the post's enormity only really struck me in the first week. No matter how much material you read to understand the post, its implications and its dimensions, those first niggles arrive when you sit down in your office for the first time. What was so different about this post? I had, prior to this, been a clinical nurse specialist for seven years, an autonomous practitioner with a caseload to manage. I had a profound sense of realisation that, despite believing myself to be prepared for such a post, I was not. I was the novice Nurse Consultant. We all start somewhere in a post, but this was different as there was no concrete framework and no designated duties to perform – just a job description and my personal expectations.

Starting in a new organisation has its advantages: to the staff working there, you are the unknown quantity, which gives you time to get to know the organisation and how it operates. It also means that you have no preconceived ideas about the areas you are to work in, and both sides initially have a clean slate. As an NTC, even a novice, you soon become aware of people's expectations of you. It is debatable whether this is due to the publicity generated by the establishment of this post (the idea of 'Super nurses') or to the discussions underlying the development of the post prior to the bid being formulated by the organisation. These expectations are, however, real and at times problematic.

It is easy to become isolated in such a post in the early days, particularly when you are new to an organisation. The induction process is invaluable as this provides an opportunity to meet the team; a well-planned induction period will allow you to meet up with the key players whom you will be working with. In the early days, I felt like a trophy, being trundled out for meetings and introduced as 'our new Nurse Consultant'. At the time, this felt uncomfortable, but looking back, it is apparent that this was useful and a key strategy at that time for people to get to know who I was and to maintain the high profile of the post.

I was in the fortunate position of being located a few doors down from another Nurse Consultant, who had been in post a few months longer than I had. Here was someone I could talk to who was in the same position. In those early days, this support was vital, and I believe that this was a mutual process that benefited us both. This form of support is highly beneficial and should be developed at every opportunity. As part of the then regional support for the Consultant posts, we met regularly with all the Nurse Consultant post-holders. From these meetings as a group of Consultants based in Teesside, we formed a clinical supervision group to assist us in our development in post. This is discussed at some length in this text, and I can only emphasise here how useful I found this and suggest that it is an important development tool for any Nurse Consultant.

Running alongside these two structures of support is mentorship. Although we will not explore mentorship here, having a mentor is another valuable and necessary tool. Mentors can, if chosen well, help you to keep the issues that you will encounter in perspective and rationally approached.

So I had gone on a voyage of discovery of my new post and the organisation in which I was employed. I had undergone induction and met many key players, both internal and external to the organisation, whom I needed to link with. I had evaluated the job description in context with the strategic needs of the organisation and government priorities, developing an action plan. I had access to regional support networks, had been asked to join the Teesside Supervision Group and had the help of a good mentor. I had re-evaluated my educational needs, changed my Master's programme and enrolled on a clinical examination skills course and a nurse prescribing course. While all this was going on, I was developing the post both internally and externally to the Trust. I had developed links nationally with Nurse Consultants for older people, supported by the Department of Health, which had in turn led to my accessing the leadership programme. I had spent time discussing the role with clinical colleagues at a variety of venues and met with the front-line staff in the clinical areas where I would be working.

While all this was happening, the clinical side of the role had still to be formalised. This would form 50% of my working time and require the use of the four key functions. Figure 4.4 reminds us of the components of the role.

From Figure 4.4, it is clear that the NTC may, as an autonomous practitioner, have a freedom that is not found in any other branches of health and social care. With this level of autonomy, there is a need to be disciplined, using action plans if necessary, to stay on track. Looking at this diagrammatic representation of the post, there is a significant problem with the post that NTCs will have to address. The vast majority of Nurse Consultants have as part of their personality, enthusiasm and a drive to succeed. This is all well and good provided that you do not let this get out of control, and as a Nurse Consultant you have to control the post rather than other people. This problem can be simply split into four areas:

- personal drive and expectations
- others' expectations
- difficulty with the word 'no'
- being under perpetual scrutiny.

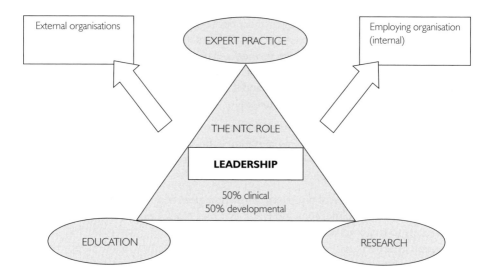

Figure 4.4   Diagrammatic representation supporting the notion that leadership is central to the NTC role

In taking on such a post, it is very easy to get caught up in the need to succeed and prove the post. The net result is that you find yourself working long hours to complete what has to be done. You find yourself involved in numerous projects, both locally and regionally, preparing presentations for conferences and attending meetings around the country that have been organised by various organisations. Your colleagues expect you to fulfil their needs, sometimes taking on roles from them that really do not fit the role of the Nurse Consultant. There is a danger that you will take on work that you know you do not have the time to complete – maybe you did not say no, or perhaps you failed to attend a meeting, only to find that a number of projects had been given to you in your absence.

This situation is, I believe, not unusual for these posts: the majority of NTCs will say that a lack of time to finish their work is a key problem area. This was a common theme in an NTC network I was involved in, and in the early days of the post, I took on far too much, resulting in overload. There is enough stress involved in starting a new role without adding to it youself just to prove that the position is successful. This affects not only your work, but also your family life. Guest et al (2001), in his evaluation of the Nurse Consultant role, cited the issue of overload caused by the size of the roles.

Finally, it is interesting that, of all the health and social care posts in existence, the NTC role appears to have been studied, researched and evaluated more than any other. At a local level, you will be formally evaluated by the organisation, which is beneficial. Informally, you will probably be evaluated by your medical and nursing colleagues, which it is probably not worth losing any sleep over. Every other week, there is both positive and negative commentary in the national professional press related to these roles. I wholeheartedly support the formal evaluation of new posts and their effectiveness, especially as these are high-profile posts, but let us not evaluate them for evaluation's sake or for the sake of interprofessional rivalry, which is pointless and can be divisive. Nurse Consultant posts are in their infancy, and the projected 1000 posts set up by 2004 has not been achieved as recruitment is proving to be problematic (Moore, 2001; Harrison, 2003). One solution is to devolve the responsibility of approving these posts away from central government to the Strategic Health Authorities. It will be interesting to see how this develops.

Such a large workload brings with it the obvious consequence that most Nurse Consultants tend not to address all four key functions at once. As each role is distinct and the post-holder unique, all posts will be developed in an indvidual way. My approach was to identify the areas where I could begin work immediately using the expert practice function, so I concentrated on inpatient areas, looking at how they ran and how evidence-based practice was delivered. Although this was, for me, an easier option, the staff initially found it quite threatening in some instances. To start this process after spending time on the ward, I found it useful to develop with the senior staff agreed ground rules for what I would and, more importantly, would not do.

While this was happening, I had time to develop the other facets of the role in a staged manner, including addressing my identified training issues. The *NSF for Older People* (DoH, 2001) became a template for my work, particularly that related to falls, and for the first 15 months I chaired the Falls Prevention Group, covering the Acute Trust and a local Primary Care Trust, and attended two other local Primary Care Trust groups to discuss falls. This eventually proved to be very time-consuming, and I eventually had to question what I was achieving. This was enough for me to realise that it was time to step out of that arena and develop other areas, my first major 'no' in post, after which it became much easier.

I have found that clinical work can cover a number of different geographical areas, in my case on two acute sites 26 km apart. I dealt with two orthopaedic wards and two outpatient clinics and medical rehabilitation wards on each site, as well as undertaking assessments in patients' own homes over a wide geographical area. Although this may not seem too much work, it is impossible to be everywhere every day – I tried, but it did not work. Deciding one's own priorities and concentrating on them may not fit with others' expectations, but at the end of the day, as the autonomous practitioner, you need to do this – after all, it is you who is doing the job.

As the clinical side of my role developed, so the need for secretarial support became evident, particularly as the outpatient clinics increased in size. It is also useful to have someone to control your appointments system, especially if organisational skills are not your strong point. An attendance at corporate meetings, aided by secretarial back-up, is essential for the profile of the post and allows you actively to contribute to the organisation's strategy developments. The appointment of a secretary also removed other administrative tasks from my daily routine, freeing up more time for my increasing clinical work.

What is the most important function of the role?

So if I had to start again tomorrow, where would I begin? Leadership is the fundamental building block of the NTC post. Associated with this must be a good understanding of yourself and how you interact with others. In the early days in post, my associate and fellow NTC within the Trust reintroduced me to the work of Covey (1989) and his framework for highly effective people (Figure 4.5).

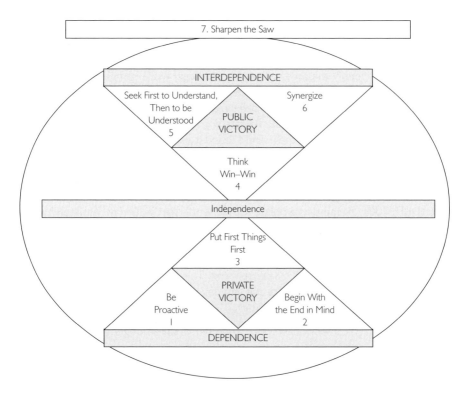

Figure 4.5   The 7 Habits of Highly Effective People (Stephen R Covey, 1989 Simon and Schuster, New York)

Covey's model has helped with my planning for the development of the post. From a personal viewpoint, the model is very similar to how I feel the NTC role develops, and having such a framework has helped this passage. The other key leadership theory that I have found useful is that of Bennis (2003), who discussed the importance of knowing your self and the world in which you operate.

Being an NTC is not for the faint-hearted or the naive. I have noticed a move towards the NTCs taking on management responsibilities for teams. Talking to individuals who have opted for this approach, I wonder where they get the time to take this on as it must impact upon some other aspect of the NTC role (Da Costa, 2002). A common answer when asking why this amalgamation has occurred is that it is only when you have management responsibility that can you truly affect changes to services. This appears to be a method to bring about rapid change using a managerial approach.

But the question of leadership needs to be considered here. Managers do not always lead, and leaders do not always manage. Are we in danger of marginalising the leadership role by taking on the management of a service? If the basis for Nurse Consultant roles was to keep practitioners in clinical practice rather than taking on non-clinical roles such as management, is this potentially counterproductive to the post, and is there a danger that the Nurse Consultant and manager roles might become one all-encompassing post? Time will tell; this may be the next development of the post, a local solution to a complex issue or a mistake. We will have to wait to see what happens and what, if any, benefits this approach offers. The NTC role is at the cutting edge of health and social care in terms of encouraging a change in practice in modern times. With the autonomy attached to this role, the NTC may not be an easy transition to adapt to, but it is definitely exciting and rewarding.

RECOMMENDED READING

Carlson R (1998) *Don't Sweat the Small Stuff at Work: Simple Ways To Minimise Stress and Conflict while Bringing out the Best in Yourself and Others*. Hodder & Stoughton, London.

Guest D, Redfern S, Wilson-Barnet J et al (2001) *A Preliminary Evaluation of the Establishment of Nurse, Midwife and Health Visitor Consultants*. A Report to the Department of Health. Kings College, London.

Harris A, Harris, T (1985) *Staying OK*. Pan, London

National Health Service Executive Trent Cancer Nurses Allied Health Professionals Advisory Group. (2001) *Nurse Specialists, Nurse Consultants, Nurse Leads: The Development and Implementation of New Roles to Improve Cancer and Palliative Care*. An Advisory Report. NHS Executive, London.

Oliver R. (2002) *Inspirational Leadership: Henry V and the Muse of Fire*. Spiro Press, London.

USEFUL WEBSITES

National Health Service Modernisation Agency Improvement Leaders' Guide (2004)
http://www.modern.nhs.uk/improvementguides/global_home.htm

REFERENCES

BBC News online network (1998) Health Nurses: We are already doing the job. http://news.bbc.co.uk/1/hi/health/166880.stm

Benner P (1984) *From Novice to Expert: Excellence and Power in Clinical Nursing Practice*. Addison-Wesley, Menlo Park, California.

Bennis W (2003) *On becoming a leader*, revd edn. Perseus Publishing, Oxford.

Butler, Nicholas Murray from http://www.brainyquote.com/quotes/quotes/n/nicholasmu125315.html

Chambers 21st Century Dictionary (2004). www.chambersharrap.co.uk

Covey SR (1989) *The 7 Habits of Highly Effective People: Powerful Lessons in Personal Change*. Simon & Schuster, New York.

Da Costa S (2002) Haunted. *Nursing Management* 9(6):11–15.

Department of Health (1999a) *Agenda for Change*. DoH, London.

Department of Health (1999b) *Nurse, Midwife and Health Visitor consultants: Establishing Posts and Making Appointments*. Health Service Circular 217. HMSO, London.

Department of Health (2001) *National Service Framework for Older People*. DoH, London.

Department of Health (2002) *Developing Key Roles for Nurses and Midwives: A Guide for Managers*. London, DoH.

Editorial (2002) *Journal of Medicine* 2, 5–6.

Guest D, Redfern S, Wilson-Barnet J et al (2001) *A Preliminary Evaluation of the Establishment of Nurse, Midwife and Health Visitor Consultants*. A Report to the Department of Health. Kings College, London.

Harker J (2001) Role of the nurse consultant in tissue viability. *Nursing Standard* 15(49):39–42.

Harrison S (2003) Health authorities to rule on Nurse Consultant posts. *Nursing Standard* 17(26):7.

Jones, P (2002) Consultant nurses and their potential impact upon health care delivery. *Clinical Medicine* 2(1):39–40.

McSherry R (2002) Developing a strategy for implementing practice development. In McSherry R, Bassett C (2002) *Practice Development in the Clinical Setting: A Guide to Implementation*. Nelson Thornes Ltd, Cheltenham.

McSherry R, Pearce P (2002) *Clinical Governance: A Guide to Implementation for Healthcare Professionals*. Blackwell Science Publications, Oxford.

Manley K (1997) A conceptual framework for advanced practice: an action research project. Operationalising an advanced practitioner/consultant nurse role. *Journal of Clinical Nursing* 6(3):179–190.

Moore A (2001) Searching for a role. *Nursing Standard* 16(8):19.

National Health Service (2004) *The Improvement Network: Connecting People with Knowledge and Innovation*. http://tin.nhs.uk/welcome

Wanless D (2002) *Securing our Future Health: Taking a Long-term View*. HM Treasury, Crown Copyright, London.

Ward M, Titchen A, Morrel C, McCormack B, Kitson A (1998) Using a supervisory framework to support and evaluate a multiproject practice development programme. *Journal of Clinical Nursing* 7(1):29–36.

Watson R (2002) Media Review: A preliminary evaluation of the establishment of nurse, midwife and health visitor consultants. *Journal of Advanced Nursing* 38(1): 105.

5 Exemplifying the nurse/therapist consultant: a practical and experiential approach

Mel McEvoy and Sarah Johnson

Introduction

As already identified in Chapter 1, patterns of health and social care are changing fast. This could be attributed to increasing patient choice, technological advances, changes in medical knowledge, consumer empowerment and shifting boundaries in the provision and alignment of services, to name but a few. This chapter assumes that what is highlighted as the new vision for health and social care in general also expects that the new role of the Nurse/Therapist Consultant (NTC) will contribute to modernising the National Health Service (NHS). The function of the NTC is beginning to emerge and establish itself in the opportunistic environment of the modernisation agenda. Although the forerunner in new Consultant posts in the NHS is nursing, many of the issues and conclusions also apply to Consultant Therapists.

In the beginning, the key functions of the role represented for many Consultants a framework of assigned areas of obligatory involvement. There is little preparation and little systematic pre-assessment of an individual's capability and capacity to succeed in these posts. For those working in this area, the terms of the functions are becoming familiar:

- expert practice
- professional leadership
- consultancy
- education and development
- practice and service development linked to research and evaluation.

Understanding what these functions meant was the first step in implementing the post for first-generation NTCs. These headings became a map of expected outcomes. A self-justifying assumption evolved that 'if I can provide evidence that I undertake work or projects in these areas, then I can legitimately state that I must be fulfilling the role'. This is an essential element of development but can, if it is perpetuated, arrest growth. By sticking rigidly to the description of the functions as outcomes, they can become an end in themselves rather than a means. These functions are the means by which the role succeeds in its purpose; they are *not* its purpose. The purpose, the ultimate outcome, for this post is the modernisation of the NHS in relation to the delivery of patient care. Modernisation is the continuous ongoing development and pursuit of excellence in health care provision based on the need of the patient.

The NTC's role is being created in the cultural context of an NHS built on a medically determined model of health as meaning the relief of illness and disease.

Within this model, nursing has lacked professional autonomy and has been situated at the bottom of the league in the hierarchy of health professionals providing a service, mainly because of its low academic base. The shape of the hierarchy was triangular and meant that patients and nurses were at the bottom. In this new era of change, this base is at the top.

This chapter will argue that a rationale and justification can be found within the modernisation documents that places nursing in general, and specifically the Nurse Consultant (and by extension the Therapist), as key players in redesigning the NHS around the needs of the patient.

THE GOVERNMENT'S IMPLICIT MESSAGE ON THE ROLE OF THE NTC

To understand the role of the NTC, it is necessary to recognise the background from which it has emerged.

Activity 5.1   *Reflective question*

NHS policy documents

Note down what you think are the key NHS policy documents that have guided and informed the development of the NTC.

Read on and compare your findings with those in the Activity Feedback on page 104.

According to Activity 5.1, seven Department of Health (DoH) policy documents have assisted with describing and expanding the nature, scope and remit of the NTC (DoH 1997, 1999, 2000a, 2000b, 2001, 2002a, 2002b).

NTCs should pursue policy documents and national standards that are underpinned by a robust nursing/therapy evidence base. These documents are useful in supporting the NTC in developing and reflecting a particular style of leadership, one that establishes direction and purpose, inspires and motivates. NTCs need to be leaders who are motivated, self-aware, socially skilled and able to work across professional boundaries. They need to be the next generation of leaders who challenge orthodoxy, take risks and learn from experience. One obstacle to this change is that nurses, and by extension Therapists, are often constrained by structures that limit development and innovation. The role is all about unlocking the potential that nurses have to offer. It is about developing their roles and the way in which they work, about creating the conditions to liberate and maximise potential. The NTC's role is an example of a new role with the potential to modernise the NHS.

NTCs must recognise that, according to the NHS Plan (DoH, 2000a), the NHS is in need of reform, and they must therefore anticipate a period of change and challenge. The aim of the reform is to redesign the health service around the patient. When asked, the public responded that they wanted staff to use new ways of working and ensure that care was patient centred. One of the problems highlighted was the lack of national standards. There was a demarcation between staff and barriers between services. The advocated vision is that the NHS must be redesigned around the needs of the patients. In Australia, the NTC role helped not only to develop inpatient consultation, but also to improve communication strategies across the health service (Dawson and Benson 1997). It becomes the NTC's responsibility to:

- help to achieve national standards inspected by a Commission for Health Inspection and Audit (CHIa)
- prescribe effective treatments endorsed by the National Institute for Clinical Excellence (NICE)
- collaborate with the Modernisation Agency
- promote the unification of the NHS and the Social Services, and develop pooled resources. In addition, contribute to the increase in the number of NTCs.

From a Consultant Therapist perspective, *Meeting the Challenge: A Strategy for Allied Health Professionals* (DoH, 2000b) forms an additional strategy for the NHS Plan, reiterating many of the points highlighted in the other documents. A priority is staff changing the way in which they work. Their focus will be on implementing protocol-based care. Leadership in these roles is critical to improving quality of care and supporting and developing staff. Leadership capacity and capability will be strengthened in three ways in the development of new Therapist roles, joining health and social care together and promoting work in partnership. The Consultant Therapist should contribute to increase fast, accessible care for those with cancer, heart disease and mental illness, and for older people, protocol-based care and health promotion in the community. The new career opportunity will help to retain experienced staff and strengthen professional leadership.

Most of the previous documents illustrated the type of work that needed to be undertaken in acute settings. In *Liberating the Talents* (DoH, 2002b), the focus of the NTC is on improvements in primary care. This document informs us that it is these primary care changes that lie at the heart of the NHS Cancer Plan. The roles must change the traditional ways of organising and delivering nursing services to a service that responds to patients' needs and wishes. The NHS Plan needs to be integrated around the needs of patients and communities. Its slogan is that patients should receive the right care, in the right place, at the right time.

NTC roles will be involved with the devolution of power and resources to the front line to give health professionals who provide the care freedom to innovate. It should increase flexibility between services and between staff to cut across outdated organisational and professional barriers. There should then be a greater diversity of service providers and choice for consumers.

In brief, it is without doubt that the NTC has the potential to facilitate and initiate change in support of the government's quest for modernisation of the NHS. To achieve the latter, it is important that NTCs familiarise themselves and their colleagues with the key policy documents, national standards and guidance. Furthermore, the familiarisation and utilisation of existing evidence originating from policy, national standards and guidance are useful aids to supporting the NTC in implementing the key elements of the role.

Activity 5.1   *Feedback*

NHS policy documents

Seven key Department of Health policy documents have emerged that have influenced the role development of the NTC:

DoH (1997) *The White Paper: NHS Modern Dependable.*

DoH (1999) *Making a Difference: Strengthening the Nursing, Midwifery and Health Visiting Contribution to Health and Healthcare.*

DoH (2000a) *The NHS Plan. A Plan for Investment. A Plan for Reform.*

DoH (2000b) *Meeting the Challenge: A Strategy for Allied Health Professionals.*

DoH (2001) *A Preliminary Evaluation of the Establishment of the Nurse, Midwife and Health Visitor Consultants.*

DoH (2002a) *Developing Key Roles for Nurses and Midwives: A Guide for Managers.*

DoH (2002b) *Liberating the Talents: Helping Primary Care Trusts and Nurses To Deliver the NHS Plan.*

DECIPHERING THE KEY FUNCTIONS OF THE NTC

This section expands on the information presented in previous chapters associated with the key components of the NTC role by explaining in detail the core functions of the role as 'experienced' by the author. What is offered are a number of insights derived from attempting to comprehend the concept of the post while undertaking the role. The key elements and function of the role to be explored are illustrated in Figure 5.1.

Expert practice

To begin with, there are many facets to the idea of 'expert practice'. Some may find the following statement obvious, but being an expert in practice cannot be equivalent to a fixed level of knowledge, skills and competencies. There are possibly several dimensions to the concept. Broadly, they may involve the individual practitioner's level of competencies in a particular speciality, influenced by the particular client group with its different degrees of complexity. It may also be influenced by the managerial and leadership development in the clinical area where the care is provided, the best evidence base available and access to such information. The clinical priorities of the particular Trust in addressing the National Service Framework (NSF) and NHS Plan may also have an effect. As all

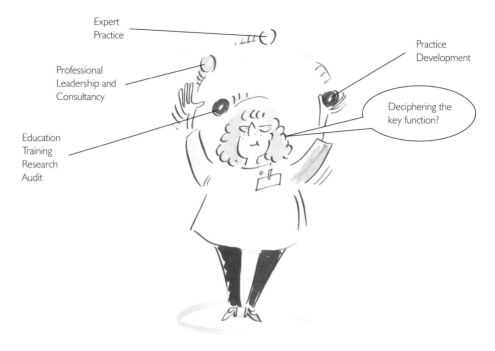

Figure 5.1   Deciphering the key functions of the NTC

these dimensions will be sources of influence, there cannot be a fixed point at which all these components are achieved.

Expert practice is therefore a process rather than a definitive and standardised function. The individual practitioner must be aware of and informed by the most relevant evidence-based approach to a particular clinical problem. He or she must be able to apply this level of skill and knowledge within the clinical area, and the clinical environment must be so constructed as to integrate this different service provision. In addition, the practitioner must be an integrated member of the team whose function and relationship is formularised and agreed. The practitioner must have both the experience in the speciality and the skills to apply an evidence-based approach. An important dimension of expert practice is to deliver the strategic outcomes identified in the NSF that is particular to the practitioner's speciality.

Let us, for example, consider Palliative Care for Non-malignant Disease. The function of expertise is to provide service provision for patients with heart failure. The NSF for Coronary Heart Disease (DoH, 2000c) requires that palliative care should be a key to providing a model of care for those individuals dying of heart failure. The expert practice dimension is an evidence-based approach to the management of symptom control in heart failure and psychological support to both carers and relatives, as well as providing open and sensitive communication in this end stage. To do this, the practitioner must work in the field and be included in the clinical decision-making process.

Another way of looking at 'expert practice' is to see it from two perspectives. The first is at a micro level. This is the level at which the individual NTC is giving actual one-to-one patient care. What is provided is an intervention based on the best evidence available and dependent on the practitioner's expertise in this field. In this context, the role is direct care within a team.

The second level is a macro perspective, at which the NTC focuses on all the elements that are involved in delivering the most effective care by a team, ward or speciality. The work involves creating 'expert practice' from a strategic perspective. The aim is to achieve the highest level of expert service provision within that particular speciality. The focus will be on training and educational provision for clinical staff, the development of care pathways and the effective application of NICE guidance in practice. Leadership development within the clinical environment aims to ensure successful change and the sustainability of new developments and initiatives. It also influences the development of the most conducive behaviour, beliefs and values within the clinical environment to promote the highest degree of patient focused care. Macro 'expert practice' involves the professional development of staff and the management of practice developments; vital to this process are critical appraisal and project management skills.

The difficulty arises when organisations adopt a superficial understanding of what is meant by '50% in practice'. It is often believed that the 50% in practice should mean the direct one-to-one patient contact, but this will limit the potential contribution of a consultant to the whole process of care. The macro explanation has greater potential to influence all the care that patients receive. It looks at care from a whole-system approach rather than an individual basis, although there is obviously a need for both (McSherry, 2004)

Professional leadership and consultancy

In this section, it is important to illustrate the breadth of influence that this role has. One way of making this point effectively is to simply describe all the groups with which post-holders collaborate. In these groups, they contribute to discussions and debates, and propose specific strategies for taking an idea or an initiative forward. It is the scope of the impact that this post can have at all levels which makes it a leadership role. In this post, the leadership function has three levels – national, network and Trust – as well as a consultancy function to a number of organisations within the locality.

At *national* level, it involves being a member of the National Nurse Consultants in Palliative Care group. There are about 10 Nurse Consultants working in palliative care in the United Kingdom. The group meets four times a year, generally twice a year at the Department of Health and is linked to the Department of Health by having one of their palliative care advisors in the group. The group discusses palliative care issues, shares good practice and developments, networks and works on collaborative projects. As a group, we offer valuable contribution to the developments happening within palliative care.

I am also a member of the National Cancer Nurse Leadership Group. This consists mainly of network lead cancer nurses and some Trust lead cancer nurses.

We make up two cohorts of 20 who participated in a leadership programme in 2000. The group's remit is similar to that of the NTCs except that there are two purposes: nurse cancer leadership and promoting nursing research in cancer.

At a *network* level, I bring these two dimensions together, being involved in the Supportive and Palliative Care Steering Group and the network lead cancer nurses group. The first group is predominately focused on delivering the NICE guidance for supportive and palliative care, whereas the lead cancer nurses group focuses on achieving the Manual of Cancer Service Standards within the centres and units that form the network. It is also committed to sharing best practice and innovation in cancer care.

At *Trust* level, I am the lead cancer nurse for the Trust as well as the NTC for cancer and palliative care. The advantages and disadvantages of joining two such roles are explained in an article on leadership by McEvoy and Mullan (2003). I lead a practice development forum with a multiprofessional membership, as well as being a member of the Cancer Strategy Team that consists of the Medical Director of the Trust, the Director of Performance Management, the lead cancer clinician and the cancer manager. All the major issues related to cancer are addressed in the team's meetings. My responsibility relates primarily to patient-centred care and professional development. This group feeds into the Cancer Steering Group, which consists of members of all the appropriate agencies, clinical governance and clinical effectiveness staff, representatives of the Primary Care Trusts (PCTs), all the lead clinicians of the site-specific cancer teams and other associated professionals involved in the delivery of care for cancer.

From a clinical perspective, I am also a member of the Specialist Palliative Care Team led by a palliative care consultant and consisting of a number of Macmillan Nurse Specialists. This attempts to incorporate the three surrounding PCTs in which these specialists are based. On a wider scale, I am a member of the Trust's Practice Subgroup and work in collaboration with two other NTC's in the Trust.

I provide a consultancy function to the three surrounding PCTs as a member of their Cancer and Palliative Steering Group. I speak for the Trust on nursing issues related to cancer and palliative care developments, and offer advice on and insight into commissioning issues. There are a number of joint collaborative projects being undertaken. I offer advice and assist in the development of the Trust's palliative care pathway, as well as offering professional advice to the Workforce Development Confederation on issues related to cancer nursing and palliative care. I am involved in promoting the significance of the NICE guidance on supportive and palliative care, and in developing a network nursing strategy. I provide leadership development to Clinical Nurse Specialists in cancer and palliative care and have links with Franklin-Covey leadership developments.

In the selection process for NTCs, the potential for leadership is top of the selection criteria. These are new posts without much of a precedent, and the NTC has to create something that did not previously exist, sometimes without support or guidance. All the individual's skills and abilities are tested within the first two years and beyond: those first two years are the ones that actually produce the pressure and problems that the individual is forced to solve.

Many authors suggest that the talent required for leadership is to see the larger actual picture and to create a vision that is compatible with the political landscape of organisations. Leadership requires an individual to see a different way of delivering a particular provision and then to enable people to see it as a solution and own the process of moving from one state to another. The art of leadership involves convincing a group that what you see as an alternative would be more beneficial.

Nursing leadership is a different type of leadership than what is generally perceived as traditional leadership. It influences organisations to develop and improve systems and approaches in order to develop more effective care for patients. Patients have to be at the heart of nursing leadership. The work is based on changing and challenging systems and processes so that they can improve care. A nurse must be concerned with guidelines, protocols, pathways, standards, single documentation and single assessment. Nursing facilitates multidisciplinary working for the sake of patients; it knows that patients will benefit if it can improve how teams work. For this reason, nurses concentrate on and influence the processes that are involved in delivering care.

This is hidden leadership, often unseen. We often view leadership as an end in itself, but when it is applied to nursing, leadership is seen as ensuring that systems function and are co-ordinated for the sake of patient care. Nursing leadership attempts critically to review approaches to care from the patient's perspective and to construct systems that relate to their needs.

Education, training, research and audit

It could be argued that each of the following functions of this post is a job in itself. Indeed, in many Trusts, these particular functions have evolved into whole departments within an organisation. In the broad description of this post, the implication is that they are a major part of the role. The difficulty lies in trying to explain how these aspects can be undertaken on top of the other aspects of the role. It suggests that this whole area is flawed with unreal expectations surrounding the post that tend to make it practically impossible to achieve. The aspects contained within my own role have educational and research components (Box 5.2).

Box 5.2   Educational and audit involvements of the NTC

- National lectures
- Associate Lecturer for the Open University
- Lecturer for the local university on health
- Lecturer within the Trust
- Involvement in training
- Involvement in research
- Undertaking audit in clinical practice

All these aspects of this function cannot be taken out of context. The educational aspect brings together the national agenda, with its application to clinical practice. The positive advertisement is that someone involved in shaping and changing the system of care teaches fellow professionals about the process.

Practice development

The term 'practice development' implies definite changes in clinical practice as a result of project work (Page, 2001). This section of the chapter will explore initiatives that are changing or have actually changed practice.

Since the post was developed, three new palliative care posts have been developed, in education, social care and health, as a result of a New Opportunity Fund Bid for palliative care for children with complex needs. A regional conference has taken place that highlights the Trust's work undertaken according to the *Manual of Cancer Service Standards* (DoH, 2000d). Within this Trust, a Practice Development Forum has been developed that supports and takes forwards development initiatives. It meets monthly and is attended by multi-professionals working in cancer. These three ideas represent the larger picture, but there are smaller practice developments that are making an impact.

This function of the role involves new ways of working. The value lies in constructing something uniquely different, in changing the system to respond to both patients' needs and the team providing the care. This is about internal change and involves ownership by members in the particular speciality. For example, the *Manual of Cancer Service Standards* (DoH, 2000d) is concerned with adding to structures and systems a new idea of patient-centred care.

Practice development must involve multidisciplinary working and in many instances also encompasses multiagency working (Ward et al, 1998; Page, 2001; McSherry and Bassett, 2002). Within this function, the difference made by the post can be measured. As with the NTC post, it has to develop where the function did not exist before. It has also to become an inherent part of the organisation. Practice development is the same process. It is the development of an idea that grows into an initiative, being owned by the organisation and over time changing the system to accommodate the new way of working. It causes a cascade of doing things differently that ultimately makes the organisation produce better outcomes of patient care.

The strength of a practice development initiative is that it should originate through direct patient and care intervention. It emerges through debate and discussion with families, in many instances because of events and situations in which the system of care is failing patients. The practice development initiative begins with an analysis and exploration of the problems and difficulties related to inadequate care. The patient and care with the NTC start the process of change. The NTC attempts, through partnership, to find a solution to the problem of a system failing patient care. The NTC knows the way through the organisational maze to enable the system and organisation to change in the light of the patient's and carer's dilemma.

Clinical governance is a key aspect of the role of the NTC. Having described the key function of the role of the NTC, it is imperative to see whether a model for the conceptualisation of the role exists, as is outlined in the next section.

THE DEVELOPMENT OF A CONCEPTUAL MODEL FOR THE NTC ROLE

The NTC role is becoming a concept within nursing, the allied health professions and the NHS that cannot be ignored. It is difficult to define a conceptual model for the role of the NTC that is based on the purpose of the post identified in the modernisation agenda and constructed around the key functions.

In broad terms, a conceptual model is a map of ideas that describes both function and purpose. There are problems with attempting to capture the map of the role as it may differ between organisations depending on the organisational needs and structures in place to support the role. The reasons for its creation and the skills of the individual in the post need also to be considered as it is a relatively new role.

Some posts-holders might perceive their role as having a strong clinical focus illustrating the 'expert practice' role, and may rarely move on to any of the other functions. Some might gradually explore the other areas as they gain confidence through their clinical achievement. Others might stretch themselves to encompass all the functions and undertake these superficially. Some posts may be accompanied by a deliberate Trust agenda, and others might leave the scope of development to the post-holder's own initiative. If this is a Trust-driven post, many of the doors will be opened, but the individual NTC may sense that he or she has become involved in managerial issues. If development is left to the post-holder and he or she is unsupported, there can be difficult struggles in gaining access to significant people and the vital decision-making mechanisms.

To help in this pursuit, Wilshaw (2004), an NTC in mental health, has begun to conceptualise the work that he does. I have chosen to use and build upon this because I recognise commonalities between my own personal experience of the post and what he describes. For the purpose of my role, I have taken what I perceive to be seven levels of intervention and defined them according to my own experience. This section is therefore closely related to the work of Wilshaw (2004) and his conceptualisation model.

Wilshaw uses two key ideas related to his model – abstraction and systemic impact – and I will describe my own interpretation of these terms here. 'Abstraction' suggests that the idea of a concept is to make an attempt to capture the essence of a particular role or function. The term 'systemic impact' is relatively self-explanatory, my interpretation being that it asks the questions, 'What does the role create that is new?, 'How is this achieved?' and 'What difference does it make?'

The real value of Wilshaw's (2004) work is that he captures in a clear way the sphere of influence and the definite areas of contact within the whole system of health care that this post must encompass if it is really going to be involved in redesigning the NHS around the patient's needs. The role of the NTC has to make its presence known in the decision-making areas of the system. Figure 5.2 shows the actual type of work in which this post must be involved. From a macro view of the role here is a way of conceptualizing seven dimensions to understanding the role:

1 'Patient care' which means actually seeing patients.
2 Mentoring staff providing clinical supervision.
3 Working with multidisciplinary teams in practice development.
4 Working with whole units or directorates and networks.
5 Working with the development of pathways, policies and protocols.
6 Working with commissioning managers in service planning.
7 Strategic partnership developments with the Strategic Health Authority (SHA) policy leads. Also the Workforce Development Confederation.

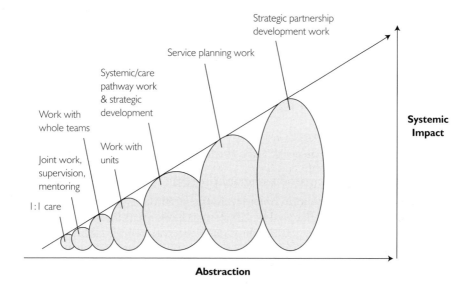

Figure 5.2 Example of a number of possible educational and decision-making contributions the Nurse Consultant could participate in under this function. Reproduced from Wilshaw (2004).

Figure 5.2 illustrates this and suggests that all these areas are the legitimate territory of the post-holder. These areas make and influence the system that delivers the care, and if the NHS system is to be redesigned around the needs of patients/clients, this is where the NTCs should be making their impact.

Figure 5.3 shows the direction of the systemic impact. All these elements of the system should be geared and focused on the quality of patient care. In this role, it is possible to bring the actual difficulties encountered in the clients' experience of care and the possible organisational difficulties directly into the arena of the SHA and Workforce Development Confederation. This is the crucial decision-making level at which change is made permanent. The whole area of abstraction is the area of influence and concern. The NTC's ability to gain access here means that patients' needs and experiences can directly influence the development of the system.

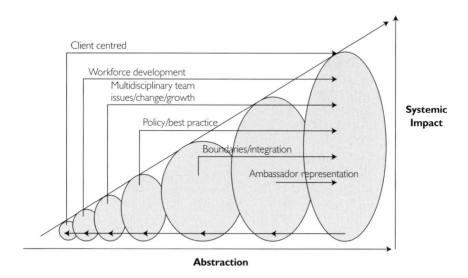

Figure 5.3   By perceiving the role in this way it is easier to conceptualise and measure its impact in the health care setting. Reproduced from Wilshaw (2004)

The initial developments of a referral process

At a certain stage in the embryonic development of the role, the NTC has to be aware of and make clear the type of service that he or she is attempting to provide and to make that service visible through a referral process. Many NTCs are working within their organisations and bringing about service developments that improve patient care. For this, it is necessary to create a coherent referral process so that the post-holder can plan and co-ordinate the difference that he or she wishes to make. The difference with this referral is that it can come from any of the seven areas that illustrate the health care provision.

I will highlight here three components of the referral process. The first consists of seven levels of intervention, from direct patient care to collaborative working with the SHAs and Workforce Development Confederation. The level of complexity grows at each level, and the skills required become more complex.

The second component covers the functions identified in the role: expert practice, leadership, education, training, research, audit and practice development. Each level may involve all the functions or simply one. The contribution or work undertaken may bring practice issues to bear on theory and policy, but central to this process is patient care.

The third component is the developmental process. A problem in the clinical area may start within one individual within a ward but, if appropriate, may require a strategic solution to fundamentally eradicate the problem. The image is one of a Russian doll representing a strategic and clinical element: an issue may start in one particular ward but ultimately inform the Department of Health. This suggests that there are many stages in changing service delivery, and the issues could be clinical and strategic.

The referral criteria for seven levels of intervention

1 **The provision of direct patient care**. The issues would be related to palliative care, for example symptom control, psychological support and ethical issues. The function would be expert practice.
2 **The provision of mentoring to the clinical staff,** clinical supervision and action learning sets based on the issue identified. It might be joint partnership in caring for a patient with a particular problem. The goal is the empowerment of staff, and the function is leadership
3 **Working with whole teams** such as multidisciplinary in the functions of leadership, education and training related to the NSFs and the *Manual of Cancer Service Standards* (DoH, 2000d). Developing a possible vision of how to collaborate and achieve the goals and standards effectively.
4 **Working with whole units** such as directorates, clinical effectiveness and clinical governance regarding policy and strategy development in order to achieve the national requirements. It could include expert practice, leadership, education, training, audit, research and practice development.
5 **Working with organisations in cross-boundary strategies** in the development of care pathways, policies and protocols. Ensuring that both primary and secondary care are effectively interfaced. This could include expert practice, leadership, education, training, audit, research and practice development.
6 **Working at network level** and with commissioning managers within PCTs. The issues would be related to cancer and palliative issues, and the role would adopt a consultancy capacity. This might involve fostering the collaboration of organisations around collective bids and initiatives such as the New Opportunity Funded Bids for projects, implementation of the NICE guidance and the *Manual of Cancer Service Standards* (DoH, 2000d).
7 **Working in strategic partnership** with the SHA, university curriculum development, Workforce Development Confederation, Modernisation Agency, CHIa and Department of Health. To this level of consultancy, NTCs will bring their experience and knowledge of the other levels so the scope of their insight is vast and crosses boundaries.

Looking at nursing or therapy from this perspective allows us to provide patients and clients with individual practitioners who are in touch with the whole system, its processes and outcomes, and are in a position to attempt to redesign the system. It is the NTC's accessibility to all these areas that provides insight into what the difficulties are. From this insight, patient-centred solutions develop. The

NTC is active in these areas to ensure that quality of care is built into the redesigned system.

CONCLUSION

In this chapter, I have tried to make sense of the role and its functions, to integrate the implications of the government documents and to explain the practical side of the role by simply stating what I do. I have also attempted to build for the future by proposing a conceptual model built into the heart of practice whose centre is patient focused but recognises that there are seven distinct ways of influencing patient care. The conceptual model is useful because it can deal with the strategic and clinical perspective, as well as the height and depth of nursing, and can acknowledge the need to change systems.

SUMMARY OF KEY POINTS

- The NTC has the potential to facilitate and initiate change in support of the government's quest for modernisation of the NHS.
- The NTC knows the way through the maze of an organisation to enable the system and organisation to change in the light of the patient's and carer's dilemma.
- The role of the NTC is becoming a concept within nursing, the allied health professions and the NHS, and should not be ignored.
- It is difficult to define a conceptual model for the role of the NTC that is based on the post's purpose. The work of Wilshaw (2004) has begun to make some inroads into developing a model for the role of the NTC that can be applied in practice.
- NTCs are working within their organisations and bringing about service developments that improve patient care. It is necessary to create a coherent referral process so that post-holders can plan and co-ordinate the difference that they wish to make. Applying the seven levels of intervention enhances this aspect of the role in practice.

CASE STUDY 5.1   APPLYING THE SEVEN LEVELS OF INTERVENTION

Mel McEvoy

Applying the seven levels of intervention provides a useful framework for exemplifying the key functions of the NTC role, as the following case study illustrates. The individual examples are practical and experiential, being based around my experiences as an NTC over the past four years.

Level 1: direct patient care

Cognitive behavioural therapy for clients with a life-threatening illness

A crucial component of palliative care is psychological support. There is evidence that cognitive behavioural therapy has proved to be beneficial with some patients with a life-threatening illness such as cancer who also have depression, low mood and anxiety (White, 2001). With several years' experience of providing psychological care to cancer patients, and having undertaken a course in cognitive behavioural therapy, I have been providing this intervention to selected patients.

Patients have been referred to me by Clinical Nurse Specialists. One particular patient suffered from depression following a diagnosis of cancer. He was a very agitated man encumbered by a great deal of suffering. Under the clinical supervision of a trained therapist, I explored over three sessions the meaning of this suffering.

The first session was awkward as this gentleman was preoccupied with his wife's health. I therefore rearranged the meeting to take place in his own house. While making my initial assessment, we sat and discussed some topics related to what the process would involve and talked about the goal focus of the sessions. At the end, I asked how valuable the session had been, and he said he was 49–51% in favour of coming again.

When we next met, we explored some of this man's feelings and negative thoughts. I explained the nature of the intervention, and at the end of the session, I asked him to rate the value of the session, to which he replied 50–60%. We had explored some deep material and set some simple goals to work towards before the next session. The gentleman went into the local hospice for respite but then acquired a severe chest infection and increased pain. After his discharge, he was admitted to an acute ward and died there a day later.

Some elements of this scenario were unsatisfactory, but it was good that the patient himself identified the positive contribution. The next stage could be to increase the skill of other professionals in delivering this type of care, which takes us to level 2.

Level 2: mentoring clinical supervision professional support

A client with Creutzfeldt-Jakob disease

The Deputy Director of Nursing asked whether I could offer professional support to a primary care team who were caring for a client with Creutzfeldt-Jakob disease. This was the first case known to the Trust. There was considerable uncertainty about the trajectory of the illness and the management of the symptom control. I contacted the surveillance unit in Edinburgh for information and insight, and completed a literature search on what constituted effective end-stage care of a patient with Creutzfeldt-Jakob disease. Based on the little available literature that there was, I created a synopsis of important nursing care points and presented them to the care team. I combined my previous skills and knowledge of palliative care with the best available evidence for the symptom management of a patient with CJD. The immediate care team and family found this helpful.

I met the client and family several times. A major ethical decision arose over the introduction of a PEG tube for his nutritional needs, and his mother needed some guidance and support. There is a lack of understanding about the end stage of this disease. The ethical arguments were that, as far as we understand, the client was dying, and the introduction of artificial administration of nutrition would not add to quality of life because of the effect of the brain disease: the client at this point was unable to speak or see and presented with signs of dementia. Insertion of the PEG tube would have been an ethical decision if drugs for symptom control could not be administered orally and if the client would have benefited from nutrition administered through a PEG tube. The question was whether he was dying of the disease or of malnutrition.

The situation was reviewed when a specialist came from the surveillance unit and recognised that the client was already in the end stage of the disease. This information was crucial to the ethical dilemmas. Based on this information, my argument changed from encouraging the possible introduction of a PEG to the fact that this would not be in the client's best interest, meaning that I had expressed two different points of view about the care of this client. I provided literature relating to ethical issues concerned with feeding and not feeding, and we had an in-depth discussion. I explained prior to the visit from the surveillance unit that one course of action would be to insert the tube, but the expert's visit provided us with more information. Clarification and explanation enabled the mother to feel that she was making an appropriate decision by not acting.

I liaised with the local hospice and obtained permission to admit the client for this end stage. I worked a few shifts in the unit and provided psychological support to the carers. He died peacefully surrounded by his family. Since this initial experience, I have provided advice and support to care teams in different parts of the country. They also found the summary of information and being informed about the potential ethical issues very useful.

Level 3: working with a whole team related to the NSF

Setting up a clinic for clients with heart failure

The NSF for coronary heart disease (DoH, 2000c) asks for a palliative care provision for patients with heart failure. After many failed attempts to explore this need with cardiologists, I discovered an opening via a geriatrician with a special interest in cardiology and heart failure.

The aim is to provide palliative care for patients in end-stage heart failure, which will take the form of a heart failure clinic. It is well known in cardiology that it is difficult to discern when a patient is in stage four of the New York Heart Failure Scale, and with drugs and treatment compliance, the patient may revert to stage three. Professionals who frequently work in this area are familiar with the cluster of symptoms. The patient may be cachexic. There will be some degree of renal impairment. It is likely that breathlessness and an accumulation of fluid in the lung will occur. Ankle and leg oedema are likely to be present, and a raised jugular venous pressure can be visible to the eye. Fatigue is generally present.

The specific aim is to offer palliative care support in end-stage heart failure. This will include good symptom control, specifically of breathlessness, and will offer psychological support to patients who may be aware of dying and wish to explore related issues. It will also attempt to establish the preferred place of care for these patients, along the same lines as a living will. The situation may well be identified as an expected death, and support is about enabling the patient and family to make a choice of where care should be provided. It will look at a close, collaborative co-ordination of care between acute and primary care. Primary care teams will need to be familiar with the end-stage management of someone with heart failure, and psychological support will be provided to carers, who will play a vital component in the management of this patient's death. End-stage care should be governed by the care of the dying integrated care pathway.

This will be a pilot project that will be researched, audited and evaluated to assess the effectiveness of the model.

Level 4: working with whole units in strategy development and implementation

Patient-centred care

Every Acute Trust in the country is assessed via a regional peer review on their compliance with the *Manual of Cancer Service Standards* (DoH, 2000d). I was asked to lead on the development of Topic One: Patient Centred Care. I gathered 12 Clinical Nurse Specialists together to decide on how we could address this issue. I also linked in with the training and development department of the Trust for their support, in conjunction with a post (Leading an Empowered Organization) leadership programme.

The strategy for achieving Topic One evolved as follows. First, I split the group into two working groups that fitted in with their clinical commitments. The Clinical Nurse Specialists were given half a day a month to work on this project. The half-day consisted of one hour on leadership development looking at the work of Covey's 'The 7 Habits of Highly Effective People' (Covey, 1989), one hour on action learning sets related to the project and a final hour on the actual project work.

The Trust has two general hospitals, the Nurse Specialists from each site being paired together. When we analysed the *Manual of Cancer Care Standards*, seven themes emerged. The need for each cancer site-specific multidisciplinary team to complete a survey of patients' experience related to the care they received. They also needed to develop site-specific patient information. Each team had to ensure that patients were involved in their own care and the decision-making process. The members of each team also had to have effective communication skills related to exploring difficult issues associated with cancer. Each team had to develop support groups, and consideration had to be given to how multidisciplinary teams function. There was a need for all projects to be related to primary care and recognise the importance of the interface. In order to achieve these projects, an educational needs assessment was undertaken of all the members of each site-specific multidisciplinary team.

The strategy was that one team would look at one aspect of the topic in depth and then share their knowledge with the other teams. The end result would be that each multidisciplinary team for breast, colorectal, lung, gynaecological and urological cancer would have achieved all these projects and thus achieve the standard. It was an important principle that although the nurses led the initiative, a key leadership function was to facilitate ownership by the whole team. The finishing line would be that the whole cancer unit would be effectively delivering patient-centred care. There were two additional milestones: a regional conference to celebrate this work followed by the collective writing of an article sharing our work nationally in a nursing cancer journal.

Stage one of the process has been achieved: each group completed the work and presented it at a conference. The next stage involves sharing each project across all the teams until every team has achieved all the initiatives. This project involved the whole unit, addressed a national requirement for the Trust and formed part of an overall strategy in preparing the cancer peer review.

Level 5: working with organisations in care pathway development

Palliative care pathway
One of the biggest challenges of pathway development has been attempting to create a palliative care pathway, initially for cancer but then for all patients with a life-threatening illness. The remit for this was enormous. A group was gathered together from Specialist Nurses from acute and primary care. An extensive search of the available literature was completed and very little found. It meant starting from the beginning.

I brought a strategic perspective to the discussions and highlighted a number of key factors that needed to be considered. I suggested that the pathway should be directly constructed from the supportive and palliative care NICE guidance: the themes in the document should highlight what the pathway should consist of.

There were two initiatives that were identified in the guidance document: the Gold Standards Framework of Thomas (2003) and the Integrated End of Life Pathway, by Ellershaw and Wilkinson (2003). I was also familiar with a new important development called the Preferred Place of Care (Storey et al, 2003). If we grouped these three initiatives together with the NICE (2004) guidance, we would then be able to formulate a pathway.

The Gold Standards are standards of care that should be delivered in primary care. They include a database of patients dying in the community, held by GP practices. The Preferred Place of Care initiative consists of asking a patient who is expected to die where he or she would like to be cared for. The answer is recorded and in one sense becomes a living will. The community staff are then trained in how best to handle acute emergencies that would in the past have warranted an admission to a Trust. A key element is the support and care of carers in terms of being prepared for the end stage of the illness. The Integrated End of Life Pathway operates at a stage in the illness when death is expected and when the patient is unable to swallow and is semi-comatose. It involves a rationalisation of medication and the availability of drugs for nausea and vomiting, agitation, pain and drying up secretions. The plan of care is expected to respond to and reflect patient's wishes. These three different initiatives should be included in the consideration of any palliative care pathway.

The success of projects often depends on how they fit in with existing and well-established policy and practice. If the new initiative is a natural progression of practice, its uptake and application will be easier. It is therefore crucial to the success of the pathway to make direct reference to these projects within policy and practice, especially that related to expected death. The question of choice of where to die and the use of the Integrated End of Life Pathway should become a part of practice and be written into policy.

This particular initiative shows the analysis and synthesis of local practice with national and government policy. It is an attempt to ensure evidence-based care and adherence to the NICE guidance, as well as to find creative ways to apply the national agenda at a local level.

Level 6: working with PCTs and commissioning managers on new developments

Transitional care

The Director of Nursing asked whether I would offer professional assistance to a child with complex needs, the family and the primary care team. Major problems began to occur when the child became too old for paediatric care and there was no comparable service in the community. There was no effective co-ordination of care but a lack of collaboration between the associated agencies. Respite and support were provided outside the area, and professionals lacked the expertise to manage both carer and child with complex needs.

The initial stage was to understand the problems and establish partnership with all the key players to together work towards possible solutions. The first major goal was to establish common standards for practice that were acceptable to the client and main carer, the primary care team, the GP, external agencies outside the area for symptom control and respite care, and the paediatric team. After some modification, an agreement of the standards was reached by all involved in the care, in close collaboration with the learning disabilities team, who understand the needs of this client group. These standards were then submitted to the university, the aim being to develop a course that would provide the skills and knowledge base to be able to achieve the required standards of care. A transitional care module was created after adding another partner to the project; this was validated by the main carer and those involved in care. In collaboration with three PCTs, a New Opportunity Fund bid was successfully obtained for the development of three transitional care co-ordinators, for education, social care and health, in each of the PCTs surrounding the acute hospital.

Managing the transitional care of children with complex needs moving through several systems of service is problematic and professionally challenging for both commissioners and service providers. Tackling the injustice of inadequate service provision for a silent minority involves redesigning the NHS and social care around the needs of the patients/clients, which is directly modernising the NHS.

In this example, all the functions of the role of NTC palliative care have been brought to bear.

Level 7: working in strategic partnership with health authority, university and workforce development confederation

Informing policy development

This particular piece of work stems from the level 6 intervention. We became aware that the concept of transitional care was difficult to appreciate. The effective management of children with complex needs is problematic: the system is constructed such that no one speciality or profession has the whole picture of the needs of this client group. This group of individuals are kept alive in special baby units and, as they survive, spend much of their time in paediatric units, with many complex problems. Some attend education, and others are cared for by social services. There is no single database for this client group within any given locality. There is often a lack of specialist input owing to the complex nature of some of these illnesses, so the greatest burden falls on the family.

Although these children may age chronologically, they do not do so physically, and in some cases never leave paediatric care. Others move on without a planned and co-ordinated approach. The common problem encountered by carers is that each organisation is unaware of what the others are doing, and no one person tends to assume overall responsibility. The crisis deepens when a client and family are moved through the system without planning. The burden and stress of this lack of co-ordination falls on the family and can easily create ill-health.

When families are vocal enough, a very expensive package of care is constructed, to be deconstructed when the child dies. This results in an expensive crisis management package. In most cases, the key carer is the expert in the care relationship, knowing every aspect of the child's behaviour. Establishing a professional relationship with someone who is both expert and parent requires a different professional approach from the traditional, authority-based one.

Working in this area, we had developed a module and created three new posts that looked at the whole of health education and social care. The motto was that if the system functioned, this group and those who cared for them would get their lives back because a system would be in place that took away the burden of having to do and find everything. We realised that not only should this module be delivered to front-line professionals, but commissioning managers should also be able to access it. It should be a part of the PCT strategy.

We presented our ideas to the policy lead for children and learning disabilities, as well as to the Workforce Development Confederation, and they were very interested in the initiative for tackling this very complex problem for all organisations. They suggested that if it worked, it would make a major contribution to solving a national problem related to this client group. These groups were discussing it at policy lead level to see whether both the education could become mainstream and the co-ordinator posts could become a priority for the Workforce Development Confederation, their establishment meaning that health, education and social care would be brought together to function as a single team. Working towards a completely different approach is to modernise and redesign the NHS and social care around the needs of the client and carer.

What are the main issues for current post-holders?

One of the key questions relates to what would constitute the best preparation for such a complex post. If the NHS is going through the phase of unprecedented change – continuous as public health care needs are constantly changing – what sort of training does an NTC require to be effective?

The NTC is not only a new post, but also a radically new way of thinking about health and social care. Health and social care professionals need a new paradigm, one that is always, and should always be, concerned with developing patient care. To ensure that this ethic remains a possibility, practitioners have some responsibility for the evaluation and construction of systems of care that drive the NHS. If we see health as the care of people with illness and diseases, our systems will be medically and technologically driven. If, however, we view health as 'liberating all human potential to the fullest degree', believing that 'health is a state of complete physical, social and mental well-being, not merely the absence of disease, illness and infirmity' (Seedhouse, 1998), this should inform our judgements. It will move the act of care given to the patient into the realm of a moral act and the upholding of a person's human rights. Health and social care should be concerned with respect for people's autonomy as a key principle of health intervention.

If health and social professionals look at the much broader picture of health institutions, this should start to remove the concept of 'patient' from the role of an ill person. Based on the core documents used in this chapter and specifically looking at the key functions of the NTC role, a high level of expertise and competency is required in this new nursing function. In my role, I am consolidating the foundation of this post by seeking out specific training and education.

I am coming into my fourth year of this post and becoming more familiar with what I am doing and the key areas and competencies that NTCs require. If we keep in mind the seven levels of intervention, it is apparent that, in order to function effectively, NTCs need continuous professional development in the key components of their role. They represent the conceptual framework of professional development underlying this post. The profile of my professional skills and competencies portfolio could look like the one presented in Box 5.3.

Box 5.3   Emerging profile and key transferable skills of the NTC

Clinical
Nurse prescribing
Physical assessment skills
Palliative care qualification
Cognitive behavioural therapy qualification

Leadership and management development
Leadership skills
Strategic planning in health and social care
Project management
Change management
Practice development

Teaching and Learning
Critical appraisal skills
Honorary lectureship status at local university
Master's level education in applied ethics

Collaboration and networking
Trust clinical governance

Associated Links with CHIa, NICE, National Cancer Team, Cancer Collaborative, National Hospice Council for Specialist Palliative Care and Modernisation Agency

---

Box 5.3 identifies a growing and maturing skills and knowledge base in many of the key components of the NTC role, but learning is continuous because I still need to develop in areas where I am lacking. These components, however, go some way towards illustrating the necessary requirements for someone in the role of an NTC in cancer and palliative care.

RECOMMENDED READING

Wilshaw G (ed.) (2004) *Consultant Nursing in Mental Health*. Kingsham Press, Chichester .

REFERENCES

Covey SR (1989) *The 7 Habits of Highly Effective People: Powerful Lessons in Personal Change*. Simon and Schuster, New York.

Dawson J, Benson S (1997) Clinical Nurse Consultants; Defining the Role. *Clinical Nurse Specialists* 11, 6, 250–254.

Department of Health (1997) *A Modern and Dependable NHS for the Next Century*. DoH, London.

Department of Health (1999) *Making a Difference: Strengthening the Nursing, Midwifery and Health Visiting Contribution to Health and Healthcare*. DoH, London.

Department of Health (2000a) *The NHS Plan. A Plan for Investment. A Plan for Reform*. HMSO, London.

Department of Health (2000b) *Meeting the Challenge: A Strategy for Allied Health Professionals*. DoH, London.

Department of Health (2000c) National Service Frameworks Coronary Heart Disease. Modern Standards and Service Models. DoH, London.

Department of Health (2000d) *The Manual of Cancer Service Standards*. DoH, London.

Department of Health (2001) *A Preliminary Evaluation of the Establishment of the Nurse, Midwife and Health Visitor Consultants*. DoH, London.

Department of Health (2002a) *Developing Key Roles for Nurses and Midwives: A Guide for Managers*. DoH, London.

Department of Health (2002b) *Liberating the Talents: Helping Primary Care Trusts and Nurses To Deliver the NHS Plan*. DoH, London.

Ellershaw J, Wilkinson S (2003) *Care of the Dying – a Pathway to Excellence*. Oxford University Press, Oxford.

McEvoy M, Mullan A (2003) Should two senior cancer-nursing posts be integrated as one leadership function? *International Journal of Palliative Nursing* 9(9): 404–410.

McSherry, R (2004) Practice development and health care governance: a recipe for modernisation. *Journal of Nursing Management* 12, 137–146.

McSherry R, Bassett C (2002) *Practice Development in the Clinical Setting: A Guide to Implementation*. Nelson Thornes Ltd, Cheltenham.

NICE (2004) Guidance on Cancer Services: Improving Supportive and Palliative Care for Adults with Cancer, The Manual. NICE, London.

Page S (2001) Demystifying practice development. *Nursing Times* 97(22):36–37.

Seedhouse D (1998) *Ethics: The Heart of Health Care*, 2nd edn. John Wiley, Chichester.

Storey L, Pemberton C, Howard A, O'Donnell L (2003) Place of death: Hobson's choice or patient choice? *Cancer Nursing Practice* 2(4):33–37.

Thomas K (2003) *Caring for the Dying at Home: Companionship on the Journey*. Oxford, Radcliffe Medical Press.

Ward M, Titchen A, Morrel C, McCormack B, Kitson A (1998) Using a supervisory framework to support and evaluate a multiproject practice development programme. *Journal of Clinical Nursing* 7(1):29–36.

White CA (2001) *Cognitive Behavioural Therapy for Chronic Medical Problems*. John Wiley and Sons Ltd, Chichester.

Wilshaw G (ed.) (2004) *Consultant Nursing in Mental Health*. Kingsham Press, Chichester.

6 THE NURSE/THERAPIST CONSULTANT: PROFESSIONAL PERSPECTIVES

Aidan Mullan

INTRODUCTION

As with other new developments within the National Health Service (NHS), the role of the Nurse/Therapist Consultant (NTC) continues to be a subject of debate. Manley (2000a), Wright (2000) and Guest et al (2001) all report that the professional views of the role are varied and that this is important when looking to the future. This chapter will describe the author's personal experiences using information obtained from his recent research project.

The study was carried out using the '360 degree approach' in order to evaluate the professional expectations and impact of the NTC role. A total of 30 semi-structured interviews took place, the data being analysed using thematic analysis. Some of the findings from this are shown in Figure 6.1. The Ward Manager identified leadership skills, the Medical Consultant brought up the issue of title, the Specialist Practitioner highlighted issues of pay and status, and the Assistant Director discussed expectations and levels of expertise. Further information is discussed later in the chapter.

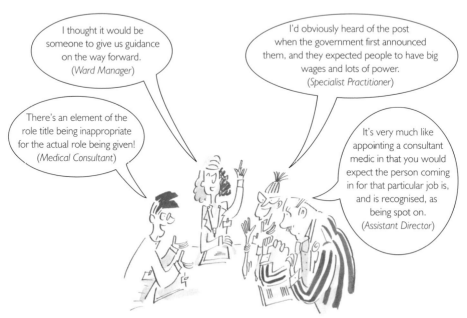

Figure 6.1 Examples of professional expectations. You would expect to see a range of the above with the NTC role.

Activity 6.1   *Reflective question*

Write down how you think other professionals perceive the NTC.

Read on and compare your findings with those in the Activity Feedback at the end of this section.

Some examples of words that you may have come up with are included in Box 6.1.

Box 6.1   Professional perspective: words and phrases associated with the NTC

For	Against
• Collaborative	• Expensive
• Strategic	• What's the difference between specialist practitioner and Consultant?
• Supportive	
• Team player	
• Clinical leader	• Conflicts
• Motivator	• Lack of clarity and understanding of the role
• Patient-centred	
• Expert	• Flexibility
• Enhanced career structures	
• Retain and recruit staff	
• Quality enhancement	

Note: You would expect to see a range of the above within the NTC role.

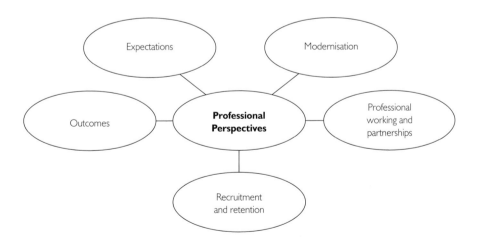

Figure 6.2   Professional perspectives: themes emerging from the research project

The themes emerging from the research project are summarised in Figure 6.2. Let us take these themes one at a time.

EXPECTATIONS

Craik (2002) and Harker (2001) state that the introduction of the NTC posts was anticipated to be a way of retaining and rewarding professionals, and this emerges as one of the themes from the research findings. The creation of the NTC post could be said to recognise the status and contribution of these professions to the NHS. These heightened expectations of the public and professionals involved could be seen to be challenging for post-holders (Harker, 2001; Da Costa, 2002; Craik and McKay, 2003). Priority needs to be seen to be given to seeking and sharing views and opinions so that ambiguities and conflicts of interest may be resolved. As Harker puts it:

> *Initial experiences suggest that the role must be flexible enough to respond to the needs of the population. Continual juggling of priorities to satisfy the requirements of the role and the expectations of the organisation has proved to be difficult.*

Responding to professional expectations is important in the delivery of the role. Essential to this is an ability to satisfy realistic expectations. Expectations of other professions may emerge from a range of sources, including professional, political, societal and individual. These can then be subdivided into two key areas of interest and concern (Table 6.1).

Table 6.1   Sources of internal and external expectations

	Internal	**External**
Professional	Professional colleagues	Professional bodies
Political	Executive/senior managers	Government
Patient/public/societal	Patient groups, carers, family members Patient advisory liaison groups	Commission for Public and Patient Involvement Voluntary/support groups
Personal	Peers	Family, friends

From Figure 6.3, it is possible to see that individual NTCs will need to develop a range of strategies in order to meet all the expectations. The figure also identifies a framework that offers a way of identifying and responding to these expectations.

The expectation–clarification exercise is about communicating with people to share and identify key aspects of the NTC role:

- *communication* – may take place through presentations, meetings, interviews and road shows
- *identification* – of issues enables the NTC to advance the role within a team or organisation
- *clarification* – is a continuing process and requires periodic discussions with others

- *support* – is a two-way process, the NTC both supporting colleagues and gaining support from the wider organisation.

The aim of this process is to enable the NTC to be accepted more quickly and easily into the organisation.

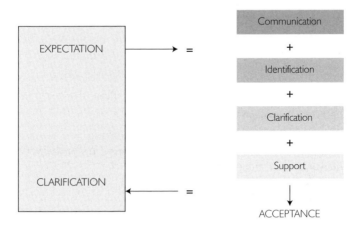

Figure 6.3   NTC framework for expectation–clarification and awareness-raising

A more robust and well-developed way of seeking and clarifying values is use of the 'values clarification exercise', a tool frequently used within practice development (Manley, 1997). The Royal College of Nursing (2002) stated that this is about:

> *developing a common shared vision and purpose. It can be used for developing a common vision about areas as different as development of role definitions, competency, or curriculum frameworks, to developing strategic direction for different purposes.*

The potential use of the expectation–clarification framework and the values clarification exercise lies in promoting partnership and collaborative working by making underlying issues explicit. These may include issues of organisation, communication, cultural differences and resource availability (Kearney et al, 2000). The benefits could be said to be improved quality of service, enhanced communication, shared working and enhanced outcomes.

MODERNISATION

This section will look at creating new ways of working, the changing workforce programme and career structures within the NHS.

The NHS plan and modernisation: creating new ways of working; changing workforce programme and career structures.

Chapter 1 explained in detail how the role of the NTC has been placed within the context of the NHS modernisation agenda. Inevitably, the successful introduction of such a role is inextricably linked with the success or failure of achieving the aims and objectives of the Department of Health (DoH) *NHS Plan*. In his foreword to the *NHS Plan* (DoH, 2000), Prime Minister Tony Blair stated:

> *This is a Plan for investment in the NHS with sustained increases in funding. This is a Plan for reform with far reaching changes across the NHS. The purpose and vision of this NHS Plan is to give the people of Britain a health service fit for the 21st century: a health service designed around the patient.*

Public consultation prior to development of the Plan showed that the public wanted to see:

- more and better-paid staff using new ways of working
- reduced waiting times and high-quality care centred on patients
- improvements in local hospitals and surgeries.

The Plan itself stated that 'In part the NHS is failing to deliver because over the years it has been under funded' (DoH, 2000). In particular, there have been too few doctors, nurses and other key staff to carry out all the treatments required. But there have also been other underlying problems. The NHS is a 1940s system operating in a twenty-first century world. It has:

- a lack of national standards
- old-fashioned demarcations between staff, and barriers between services
- a lack of clear incentives and levers to improve performance
- overcentralisation and disempowered patients.

The number of NTCs will significantly increase within the next 5 years. It is anticipated that these far reaching reforms will result in:

- direct improvements for patients
- reduced waiting times as more staff are recruited
- treatment of cancer, heart disease and mental health services – thus care in the conditions that kill and affect most people will improve
- the *NHS Plan* bringing health improvements across the board for patients, but for the first time there will be a national inequalities target. The Department of Health is presently reviewing what actual benefits to patient care have been achieved since the introduction of the *NHS Plan*. Figures 6.4 and 6.5 show that major tangible benefits to date have been a reduction in inpatient waiting times and a reduction in death rates from circulatory disease.

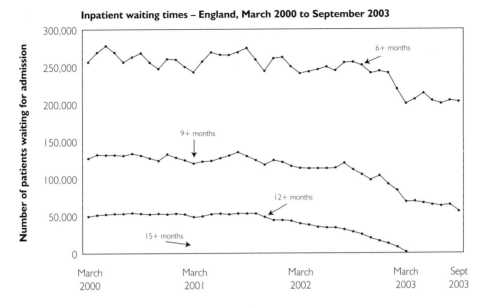

Figure 6.4   Inpatient waiting times (Adapted from Department of Health (2003) *Chief Executive's Report to the NHS*)

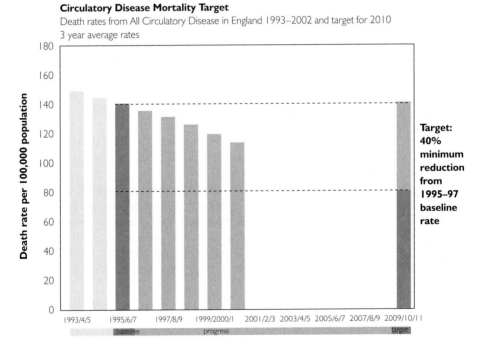

Figure 6.5   Death rates from circulatory disease (Adapted from Department of Health (2003) *Chief Executive's Report to the NHS*)

The introduction of the NTC role has in some part contributed to the reductions seen in Figures 6.4 and 6.5. In many instances, the NTC has taken the lead role in developing integrated care pathways and/or redesigning services to enable greater capacity and demand management, thus reducing waiting times for inpatient treatment (Harker, 2001; Packham, 2003). In some instances, the individual has taken on the Clinical Team Leader role, although this clinical leadership function is not always supported and valued. This echoes findings from the study, in which an Assistant Director of Nursing said, 'The nurse consultant has had a clinical lead in each of the directorates but not necessarily a clinical lead who has owned that clinical responsibility. A Nurse Specialist commented, 'I think the NTC has got to lead by example.'

It is evident that organisations and indeed individuals need to identify support mechanisms and leadership/personal development programmes to realise the NTC's leadership potential (Haworth, 2000). Harker (2001) has reported that 'The leadership function of the Nurse Consultant [Therapist] is integral to all aspects of the post, which must influence service development and clinical practice at a local and national level.' To ensure clinical and transformational leadership development for NTCs working within the NHS, it is imperative that existing managers/executives support these positions. Support within the context of leadership development is about creating the right culture and working environment that fosters and nurtures new ways of working and practice development. As Haworth (2000) puts it:

> A new management culture must appoint Nurse [Therapist] Consultants and, stand back, it has always been that way with medical consultants. The support Nurse [Therapist] Consultant's need should not be substituted for dictatorial methods.

The title of the NTC is 'not exclusively reserved for the medical profession, but is already found in a variety of other industries' (Wright, 2000). However, Castledine (1999) purports the idea that unless these issues surrounding perceptions and quality are addressed, the nurse could by extrapolation be viewed as a mere extension of the doctor's role, with such devastating consequences as to not be regarded as experts in practice by the public.

To avoid misconceptions and to promote the leadership aspect of the NTC role, both the organisation and the individual need to prepare themselves by devising and delivering a robust preparation, implementation and evaluation strategy. This strategy should form the basis for pre- and post-interview selection, role clarification, setting parameters, organisational vision and factors, getting started and involved, raising awareness and implementing and evaluating the role (Guest et al, 2001).

In short, the NTC role demonstrates the opportunity for modernisation, quality enhancements and delivering the *NHS Plan* and, through clinical and transformational leadership, challenges and creates opportunities to liberate the nursing and allied health professions in the future. Liberation only comes with the support and backing of colleagues, professionals, the public and the NHS to move forward and change. Changing cultures, working environments, clinical practices, organisational services and perceptions is complex and challenging, demanding time and investment. 'The role of leadership in achieving cultural change is almost indisputable, with successful leadership being defined as the ability to bring about sustained change' (Manley, 2000b). A further key enhancement to leadership development and the success of the NTC seems to be the promotion of professional working and partnerships between individuals and organisations, for example the acute/community/primary care/social services.

PROFESSIONAL WORKING AND PARTNERSHIPS

The NTC can provide the conduit required to enable this effective partnership working for the benefit of patients. There are examples from the study of where this is most definitely the case:

The nurse consultant fitted in the team very well – in terms of a team and a family. The family we were working with highlighted the needs and we used that experience working together practically to inform and develop the actual service. (Principal Manager, Learning Disabilities)

The Nurse Consultant fits into the team very well, I must say; it gives us the support as well from the nursing point of view that at least there is someone senior to keep an eye on that and take this forward. What he has done, or what we have done collectively, is that we do multidisciplinary team meetings. (Consultant Orthopaedic Surgeon)

We use the Nurse Consultant quite a lot as a support teacher, and I think he works well as part of the team with the doctors and the nurse because we all know him and kind of get on with him and have good rapport. (Staff Nurse, A&E)

This notion of professional working and partnership building and/or facilitation seems to be about empowering professionals and patients to take responsibility for their own health needs and/or professional development, this being regarded as a important aspect of the NTC role: 'I have helped to integrate health and social care services and to empower people to take responsibility for their own health. This is because the principles of patient participation are integral to the [post]' (Packham, 2003). Unfortunately, professional working and partnerships have not been consistently evidenced:

I'm not sure the Nurse Consultant fits into the team! I think, I don't know what it is about nursing, but we're very critical of anything and everybody and, I don't know, I feel we're a bit..., we don't like the best in people, we're always looking for the worst if you like, or looking for the shortfall instead of looking for good things. (Nurse Specialist)

There are examples of NTCs actively contributing to the reduction of death rates from circulatory disease and indeed to the wider National Service Framework (NSF) for coronary heart disease. Once again, there are examples of them leading the development of integrated care pathways and in some instances utilising their clinical skills to contribute to the reduction of door-to-needle times for the administration of thrombolysis treatment after a myocardial infarction. Issues, however, do arise, as can be seen from colleagues' comments:

> *The Nurse Consultant has quite a difficult role in trying to sort of define problems and tackle ways round it, one of them being thrombolysis by the paramedics, which is an up and coming thing. (Staff Nurse, Coronary Care)*

> *The Nurse Consultant has physically helped make improvements towards emergency heart attack patients coming into A&E and being thrombolysed quickly and according to the National Service Framework. Three years ago when the framework came out we just weren't achieving the standard. (Senior Analyst)*

It may be questionable whether this is a practice that is relevant to the role of the NTC or something that other practitioners, for example Specialist Clinical Nurses, could and should be undertaking. NTCs are, however, contributing to other NSF initiatives and their predecessor, the Cancer and Palliative Care Plan. Indeed, many have been appointed to roles specifically developed with the various frameworks in mind, enabling a more standardised approach to the delivery of care. Their contribution is, however, often either limited or sometimes not fully recognised:

> *We're still as a department certainly quite unclear what the Nurse Consultant role is, although he/she comes and does some teaching for us around the National Service Framework in coronary care and thrombolysis, which was their main role at the time. I'm not quite sure what else they do within the Trust. (Senior Sister, A&E)*

> *I suppose, I know, there's more to the job than just what people see on the shop floor, but the nurses don't feel like they've seen them as much and I think that's because that's their world. (Nurse Specialist)*

Part of the problem seems due to individuals attempting to or being expected to undertake in equal parts the four functions of the NTC role, as described in previous chapters:

> *The role was defined that there would be a split between clinical and the education, research role, but there had to be a powerful clinic set-up for the person who had the credibility. (Assistant Director of Nursing)*

> *Certainly for the department, our expectation was that the Nurse Consultant would work two and a half days clinical within the department, and then the other two and half days would be spent in research and sort of doing updates with staff, and doing some work with the university. (Senior Sister, A&E)*

In some instances, NTCs are also being asked to work across large professional and organisational boundaries. It is clear that this is both unrealistic and unreasonable, the consequence being role overload.

I think the Nurse Consultant has found it difficult at times to balance the workload. If you're heart's really set in one area of doing research work, having a caseload, and then you're expected to be top lead, a function for a whole site, that's a tall order. (Nursing Director)

It is evident that the major early success attributable to the *NHS Plan* has been an improvement in access to health care services. In January 2004, Sir Nigel Crisp, Chief Executive of the NHS, stated, when addressing NHS leaders as part of a national consultation exercise on the *NHS Plan* and future investment priorities: "The NHS has to move from the Traditional 'Physician Centric/Sickness Care Model' to a more effective 'Chronic Care Model'" (Figure 6.6).

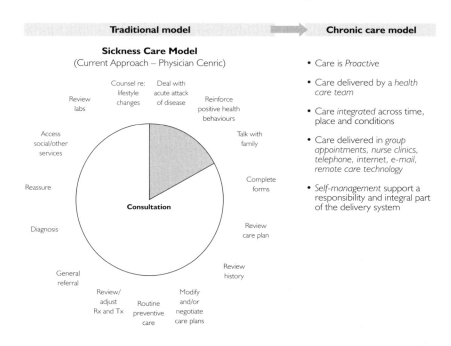

Figure 6.6 Sickness care model versus chronic care model (Adapted from Beasely C and Dowse C (2003) *Chronic Disease Management* PowerPoint presentation, Modernisation Agency, NHS

The evidence from the research would suggest that the areas in which NTCs have made most impact, albeit limited, are similar to those attributable to the *NHS Plan* and the NSF. Examples of this have been echoed by colleagues:

Well, the things that have improved are that we didn't actually have a proper system for giving thrombolysis and we now do. (A&E Consultant)

The benefit is that basically you're not unnecessarily bringing elderly people into hospital, and it frees up our clinical commitments so that we can see other patients. So in that way it has lessened our workload, but at the same time I think it has improved the care in the community. (Consultant Orthopaedic Surgeon)

The NTC should, however, have a major role in enabling the shift from a 'physician-centric, sickness care model' to an effective 'chronic care model', as highlighted in Figure 6.6. The identified components of an effective chronic illness approach are:

- effective registers and integrated records
- evidence-based care pathways
- self-care/self-management – with information and support
- an active management of at-risk patients
- primary/secondary/social care co-ordination.

The challenge for NTCs lies in creating a model of care/intervention that both complements medicine and enhances the postion of the role. Early indicators seem to suggest that the best way forward is through shared working practices that complement 'areas of working with substantial overlap between role emerges as a more effective model of service delivery' (Guest et al, 2001). Despite the enormous potential to be expected from harnessing professional working and partnerships, a perceived benefit of NTC posts relates to whether they enhance working patterns and career structures for the professions, a debate that is identified in the next section.

RECRUITMENT AND RETENTION

One of the key reasons for the introduction of the NTC role was to provide new career opportunities to help retain experienced staff within the NHS. Guest et al (2001) discussed the problem of role ambiguity and overload.

I think we all thought it would be more ward based, you know; … maybe it would be sister level or just above. We didn't realise it was going to be quite so academic. (Ward Sister)

It's quite an intensive role, and with everything else I think there was a potential for overload there. (Assistant Director)

Table 6.2 displays a wide range of views that have been expressed from members of staff of both hospital and university. These include the importance of:

- a clear job description
- co-operative working practices
- clarification of expectations
- support and mentorship
- being a bridge between the health service and the university.

Table 6.2 Key factors for success Key factors for success

Key factors for success	Rationale	Potential impact	Quotes substantiating these factors
Involvement and Inclusivity	To ensure that during the consultation process pre- and post-interview/selection and throughout the commencement of the position, the post-holder and employing team involves and includes relevant stakeholders	Reduces ambiguity, provides clarity of the role and person specification Provides an opportunity to demystify the role and responsibility of the post Enables and encourages the post-holder and other individuals to discuss the role. Provides a good opportunity to market the post	'The Trust board did not consult me or give me any information.' 'I received no information or was consulted about the role and its development' (*Two Consultants*) 'Nothing about the role, nothing about the sort of person who might be in it' (*Ward Sister*) 'Nothing about the role; the [Nurse Consultant] just appeared' (*Nursing Team Leader*) 'The role was not discussed with me; it was developed by the nursing hierarchy' (*Assistant Director*)
Informing	To resolve the issues regarding inadequate information-giving and awareness-raising in relation to the role	Reduces misunderstandings and provides a mechanism for sharing and disseminating information about the role	'I had heard about the posts in the nursing press: the people [Nurse Consultants] would get big money and have a lot of power; did not get any information from the Trust' (*Nurse Specialist*) 'Did not access or get information from the Trust; thought the role would be for a specialist helping the work of the Trust' (*Director*) 'I have read very little about this job. He comes here but there is not much information available about him' (*Staff Nurse*)
Role expectation –clarification	To address concerns or factors relating to the role's scope, purpose and remit	Ensures that the post-holder, professional colleagues and public become familiar with the purpose and remit of the post	'To take decisions about treatment programs for patients and also to train individuals and develop education and research packages' (*Assistant Director*) 'Expected he [the Nurse Consultant] would work two days in clinical practice and spend the rest of the time doing research and working in the university' (*Senior Sister*) 'I expected to see them running their own clinics and nurses would seek their assistance instead of the junior doctor. They would also teach about research and stuff like that' (*Student Nurse*)
Role attributes/ parameters	To clarify the remit of the post	Promotes teamworking by ensuring that the boundaries and parameters of the post are understood	'He's got knowledge from different backgrounds but he is a specialist so you can use him for advice; he listens to us and he gets to go to all the meetings to give our point of view' (*Staff Nurse*)

Table 6.2 *continued*

Key factors for success	Rationale	Potential impact	Quotes substantiating these factors
		Prevents role and professional conflicts between and within the profession and other professional groups	'His availability is very compromised with his current responsibilities, because he has to be available for patients, staff and the management' (*Senior Educationalist*) 'He has the remit to facilitate five clinical sessions and five educational sessions and should have a high profile demonstrating leadership skills, working in the multidisciplinary team and contributing to the Trust strategy. I don't think he has managed to achieve this; he is too willing to be pulled in too many directions' (*Director*)
Manageability/ diversity	To offset expectations that the person in role would facilitate in an academic role within the university and contribute to education and learning in practice	Demonstrates the uniqueness of the post-holder and diversities in role and responsibilities	'Someone with expert knowledge who would educate us and help us within developments. They have an educational role and a research role with the university' (*Staff Nurse*) 'Give guidance and education to staff, access research for us from the university and be a middleman to support change' (*Ward Manager*) 'Pressure from the Trust has pushed them into to many roles. They should be educating staff in all clinical areas and bringing information about research from the university, but they don't fulfil this because they are involved in too many projects' (*Primary Care Facilitator*)
Support	To contraindicate perceptions that these posts are unsupported	Encourages the post-holder to settle and engage with the role Ensures a more productive and successful role	'A very good induction programme and some secretarial support has helped' (*Medical Director*)

OUTCOMES

The challenge for NTCs, professional bodies and employers lies in establishing the effectiveness of these new posts. Read et al (1999), Reynolds et al (2000), Manley (2000a, 2000b) and Guest et al (2001) state that evaluation of the NTC role provides opportunities for capturing immediate feedback through a diverse set of measures. This will be useful in planning for future developments. As discussed earlier, the introduction of targets, such as those aimed at cutting waiting lists and reducing morbidity, are proving successful. Future plans may then be aimed at addressing other key chronic conditions for the health service.

CONCLUSION

The research study produced some very interesting findings that have helped to clarify the issues surrounding the introduction of the NTC role. Success has already been achieved in some key areas, and as the number of these posts increases, it is hoped that the NTCs' role will be fully recognised as they become members of a harmonious and effective team.

Activity 6.1 *Feedback*

Professional perspectives of the NTC are diverse and varied. Several themes are emerging which demonstrate the perceived activities undertaken by the NTC. These actvivities are primarily centred around: modernisation of the NHS, improving professional working, partnerships, the recruitment and retention of staff and the patient's/clinical outcomes.

SUMMARY OF KEY POINTS

- Expectations should be prioritised for the NTC.
- The impact of the NTC on service delivery and outcomes needs to be assessed.
- A clear job description and preparation for the introduction of an NTC post are necessary.
- NTC posts linked to governement priorities have proved successful.
- There needs to be some method of evaluating the impact of the NTC role.

RECOMMENDED READING

Craik C (2002) Consultant therapist – are you prepared? *Therapy Weekly* 13:8
Harker J (2001) Role of the nurse consultant in tissue viability. *Nursing Standard* 15(49):39–42.

REFERENCES

Castledine G (1999) Review of the statutory bodies: five into one may go. *British Journal of Nursing* 8(4):266.

Craik C (2002) Consultant therapist – are you prepared? *Therapy Weekly* 13:8.

Craik C, McKay EA (2003) Consultant therapists: recognising and developing expertise. *British Journal of Occupational Therapy* 66(6):281–283.

Da Costa, S (2002) Haunted! *Nursing Management* 9(6):11–15.

Department of Health (2003) *Chief Executive's Report to the NHS* DoH, London.

Department of Health (2000) *The NHS Plan. A Plan for Investment. A Plan for Reform.* HMSO, London.

Guest D, Redfern S, Wilson-Barnett J et al (2001) *A Preliminary Evaluation of the Establishment of Nurse, Midwife and Health Visitor Consultants.* A Report to the Department of Health. Kings College, London.

Harker J (2001) Role of the nurse consultant in tissue viability. *Nursing Standard* 15(49):39–42.

Haworth S (2000) New management culture in the new NHS. *Nurse Management* 7(3):16–18.

Kearney N, Miller M, Sermus W, Hoy D, Vanhaecht K (2000) Collaboration in cancer nursing practice. *Journal of Clinical Nursing* 9(3):429–435.

Manley K (1997) A conceptual framework for advanced practice: an action research project operationalizing an advanced practitioner/consultant nurse role. *Journal of Clinical Nursing* 6(3):179–190.

Manley K (2000a) Organisational culture and nurse consultant outcomes. II. Nurse outcomes. *Nursing Standard* 14(37):34–38.

Manley K (2000b) Organisational culture and nurse consultant outcomes. I. Organisational culture. *Nursing Standard* 14(36):34–38.

Packham (2003) Changing direction. *Nursing Standard* 17(36):58–59.

Read S, Lloyd Jones M, Collins K, McDonnell A, Jones R (1999) *Exploring New Roles in Practice Implications of Developments within the Clinical Team (ENRiP).* DoH Report. Sheffield University, Sheffield.

Reynolds H, Wilson-Barnett J, Richardson G (2000) Evaluation of the role of the Parkinson's disease nurse specialist. *International Journal of Nursing Studies* 37:337–346.

Royal College of Nursing On Line (2002) Practice development processes, outcomes, evaluation and references/tools for use values clarification. http://www.rcn.org.uk/resources/practicedevelopment/practice_toolsphp

Wright LJ (2000) Issues influencing neonatal nursing practice: inspiration or limitation. *Journal of Neonatal Nursing* 6(3):82–87.

7 THE NURSE/THERAPIST CONSULTANT: EXECUTIVE AND MANAGERIAL PERSPECTIVES

Wendy Morrison

INTRODUCTION

Nurses [and by extension Allied Health Professionals] need to be all that they can be. (Dr John Reid, Secretary of State for Health, 2003)

This chapter describes a managerial perspective of the journey from the first brief mention of Nurse Consultants in June 1998 through the development of policy and its implementation up to the end of 2003. It describes a range of responses to the new posts from the health professions, and the establishment of the role in nursing, together with some of the opportunities the role affords. It sets out the evolution of the Nurse/Therapist Consultant (NTC) through a period of rapid and extensive change and investment in the National Health Service (NHS) to a point at which the possibilities for this expansion of nursing, and by extension health and social care, are starting to be realised.

In order to provide an executive and managerial perspective of the NTC, it is imperative to outline in sequence the events and people associated with the evolution of the post, for example policy-drivers, supporters and opponents of the role, and potential of the NTC in the future. To this end, this chapter depicts the sequence of events, systems and processes that need to be or are in place to ensure that the NTC post achieves its potential.

Activity 7.1 Reflective question _____

Highlighting the main policy-drivers, supporters and opponents of the NTC role in the future

Write down what you see as the main policy-drivers, supporters and opponents that will affect the role of the NTC in the future.

Read on and compare your findings with those in the Activity Feedback on page 141.

The main policy-drivers, supporters and opponents of the role of the NTC for the future seem be associated with the ways in which the posts were introduced. From Activity 7.1, it would appear that minimal advice and guidance, through peer consultations and reviews with existing health and social care professionals, professional organisations or higher education organisations, was sought by the government. The culmination of this initial minimalist approach to the three 'C's' – communication, consultation and collaboration – has resulted in a mixed reception both within and between the professions. By taking a sequenced approach to presenting the executive perspectives and the views of the NTC posts, a more balanced understanding of the potential and opposition to these posts may emerge in the future. To begin this process, Table 7.1 illustrates a sequenced approach to presenting the executive perspectives of the NTC.

Table 7.1   A sequenced approach to presenting the executive perspectives of the NTC

Phases	Issues to consider
1) Evolution	– Launch of the role – Key policy documents
2) Recruitment and selection	– Regulating of implementation – Assessment of proposal
3) Introducing the NTC	– Reactions – Support
4) Establishing the impact of the NTC	– Agenda for change – Qualifications – Future opportunities

Table 7.1 emerged following a review of the key issues and policy documents associated with the introduction of the NTC role. It would appear that a phased approach outlining the evolution, recruitment and selection, introduction and potential impact of these roles emerges as a possible way in which to demystify the NTC. This chapter therefore presents each of these phases and issues to consider within each phase.

EVOLUTION OF THE NTC

To understand where and why the NTC was introduced into the NHS, it is essential to explain and explore where the term evolved, how the role was launched and the key policy documents underpinning the posts.

The launch of the Consultant role

The first public indication of a proposal for the creation of Nurse Consultants (and therefore Therapists) was made by Tony Blair, Prime Minister, in a speech to the Nurse '98 Awards ceremony on 8 September 1998 (DoH, 1998a). In this speech, reference was made to the results of a recent national consultation that the Government had undertaken to inform a new strategy for nursing (DoH, 1998b). Tony Blair spoke of how the consultation had revealed a widespread view of the need to strengthen clinical leadership, to develop challenging new roles and to improve career pathways and opportunities for clinical nurses. The Prime Minister announced that he would be asking Frank Dobson (then Secretary of State for Health), 'to look, with the professions, at introducing some nurse consultant posts with the same status within nursing, that medical consultants have within their profession' (Department of Health 1998a).

The national strategy for nursing – *Making a Difference* – was launched in July 1999 (DoH, 1999a). In the strategy, the role of the new Nurse Consultant was set out in some detail, thereby firmly establishing the role within government health policy and positioning it within the nursing career framework of the new nursing strategy.

The strategy made explicit the expectations of the Department of Health and provided clear signposts for the expansion of the role of the nurse in extending choice and helping patients to exercise choice.

Activity 7.1   *Feedback*

Highlighting the main policy-drivers, supporters and opponents of the NTC role in the future

By taking a phased approach to viewing the sequence of events and issues culminating with the introduction of the NTC, it is possible to illustrate that these posts originated and evolved from a combination of several important policy documents and from demands made by the public and professionals themselves.

Introducing the policy

> *Consultant Nurse, Midwife and Health Visitor posts will be established in the NHS to help improve quality and services; to provide a new career opportunity to help retain experienced and expert nurses, midwives and health visitors who might not otherwise stay in practice; and to strengthen professional leadership. (DoH, 1999a)*

Making a Difference (DoH, 1999a) identified that although the context of care was changing, nurses were often constrained from taking a proactive approach to responding to these changes. A number of factors were cited that were considered to have limited development and innovation in nursing, and here the link was made to an outdated clinical grading system. It was felt that this system had imposed glass walls and ceilings on career planning and progression, and had created a situation in which the most expert nurse leaders had little alternative but to leave clinical practice for management or education if they wanted to earn a higher salary.

The NHS Plan (DoH, 2000b) committed the government to the development of 1000 Nurse Consultant posts by 2004. The growth in their number during the first year of the development was substantial, the figure reaching 451. This growth was particularly impressive as earmarked funding was not allocated for the development, early posts instead being funded from within existing revenue allocations. The journey from policy to reality has proved to be eventful, particularly for the early pioneers of the Nurse Consultant role, and it is clear that, in some areas, the development of the first Nurse Consultants depended on the unswerving support, enthusiasm and persuasive powers of key nurse, medical and managerial leaders.

The introduction of Nurse Consultants was viewed by many as clear evidence of the government's intention not only to place nurses at the centre of its agenda for change, but also to strengthen the career prospects and pay progression of nurses. Although many were enthusiastic and supportive of the development, some viewed it as a threat. The reaction from the health community to the initial announcement of Nurse Consultants in 1998 was fairly muted, but when the proposal became government policy and featured strongly in *Making a Difference* (DoH, 1999a), the following year, a much more robust response was seen.

Having outlined where the NTC post originated, how it was launched and the key policies supporting its case, it is important to demonstrate what advice and guidance was put in place for recruitment and selection.

RECRUITMENT AND SELECTION OF NTCS

To ensure some degree of equity, parity, equality and opportunity in the recruitment and selection of NTCs, systems for regulating the implementation and assessment of proposals were introduced in the advice and guidance produced by the Depatment of Health.

Regulation of implementation

Definitive guidance for the establishment of and appointment to the first nurse, midwife and health visitor Consultant posts soon followed the launch of *Making a Difference*, being contained in health circular HSC 1999/217, issued by the Department of Health on 25 September 1999 (NHS Executive, 1999a).

This health circular made it clear that the Department of Health would be playing a key role in the process to establish Nurse Consultant posts. Regional offices were charged with ensuring that proposals were robust, that the approach was broadly consistent across the NHS and that local innovation and experience of the process was shared. In undertaking this process, regional offices were required to assess proposals against the comprehensive list of considerations for establishing new roles that had been set out in *Making a Difference*. Regional offices convened multiagency/multiprofessional assessment panels to consider and assess proposals submitted by potential employers. All proposals deemed by regional panels to have met these considerations were then submitted to the Department of Health for ministerial approval.

This process, which continued to be followed until March 2003, was considered by some Executive Directors of Nursing to be unnecessarily bureaucratic. Others expressed a view that the provision of such a robust process ensured that the principles for new Nurse Consultant posts, as set out in HSC 1999/217, were upheld and as such helped to ensure the integrity of the Nurse Consultant role during its early development.

Although both views are valid, the need for consistency of approach and assessment remains an issue for Strategic Health Authorities (SHA), who from April 2003 have had the responsibility for approval. Indeed, many SHAs have put in place processes similar to those employed by the Department of Health, a number of them, such as those covering Yorkshire, adopting a joint approach to approval in an attempt to strengthen the quality of the process.

The original guidance (NHS Executive, 1999a) set out an ambitious time frame for the establishment of the first tranche of nurse, midwife and health visitor Consultants with a request that proposals to establish these new posts be submitted to regional offices by 14 November 1999. This gave six weeks' notice to Trusts and health authorities for them to produce comprehensive proposals and business cases, which identified agreed funding sources and demonstrated consultation with partner organisations. Astonishingly, 48 proposals were submitted within this time scale in the Northern and Yorkshire region alone, and 36 of these received ministerial approval.

Assessment of proposals

The content and presentation of the first tranches of proposals received by regional offices varied, which was not surprising seeing that no template had been issued for the design of submissions. In terms of presenting the description of the role, the most popular format followed the headings contained within Annex A of HSC 1999/217 (NHS Executive, 1999a), outlining the four key functions of the role, namely:

- an expert practice function
- a professional leadership and consultancy function
- an education, training and development function
- a practice and service development, research and evaluation function.

Annex A also described how the content of each function might vary from post to post but made a clear and important statement that 'posts must be firmly based in nursing, midwifery and health visiting practice and evidence of working directly with patients, clients or communities for at least 50% of the time available'.

The paragraph containing this statement proved to be one of the most crucial in the assessment process and enabled assessment panels clearly to define the differences between those posts which are clearly nurse, midwife and health visitor Consultant posts because of the clinical element, and those which are not (but could be more appropriately described as clinical manager posts).

During the year 2000, the first 12 month period of implementation, more than half of all proposals rejected by panels for the Northern and Yorkshire region were refused because they failed to provide sufficient evidence that at least 50% of the time of the new role would be dedicated to clinical practice. Proposals have continued to be rejected by assessment panels because of a failure by proposing organisations to provide sufficient evidence of inclusion of this key component of the NTC role. During 2003, 30% of proposals rejected by three SHAs that were former part of Northern and Yorkshire region were rejected for this reason. This factor alone supports the case for a continued robust assessment process for the establishment of new NTC posts.

In short, despite the emerging differences of opinion relating to the level and amount of advice and guidance that was distributed to support the recruitment and selection processes of the NTC, the future developments for NTC posts are dependent upon ensuring that advice and guidance is set, followed, reviewed and amended so that these posts will continue to evolve and so that the right person is recruited for the right post.

INTRODUCING THE NTC

As already mentioned, the number of NTCs is expected to increase over the next couple of years, making it imperative to learn from the experiences of the early occupiers, implementers and evaluators of these roles. So what have the reactions to these roles been, and how have they been supported?

Reaction to the role

Many nurses (and indeed health and social care professionals) viewed the development of the Nurse Consultant role as a real prospect to put patients at the heart of the care process and as an opportunity to meet previously unmet health needs and service needs. This view was shared by some medical staff, health service managers and commissioners, who also felt that some services failed to meet the needs of patients, often at crucial points in their illness. New roles were designed and tailored to fill service gaps, and multiagency teams often undertook the work, with nurse leaders and medical staff engaged and working together.

Early evidence of this joint approach is reflected in the degree of innovation seen in proposals for the new posts, particularly during the first year. Many excellent examples are available of a wide variety of new roles. One impressive example was seen in the successful submission from Sunderland Royal Hospitals NHS Trust. This proposal was for a Nurse Consultant in End Stage Renal Failure, to manage all aspects of care for a defined caseload, the post-holder receiving referrals from and making referrals to medical consultants. An important feature of this proposal was the level of support from the relevant medical consultants for a role designed to provide expert nurse consultancy in an area of care previously viewed by many to have a number of inadequacies.

Opposition

Following the announcement of the development of Nurse Consultants, many in the NHS were excited by the potential for this new role and the improvements it heralded for patients, carers and staff, and were supportive of its implementation. The announcement also produced some less-positive reactions, particularly from some members of the medical profession, some nurse specialists and some managers.

Medical opposition

The negative response from some doctors seemed to have less to do with the new role of the Nurse Consultant and rather more to do with the title. A series of articles and letters appeared in the medical press that expressed views ranging from mild amusement that nurses should be granted the title of consultant, to extreme outrage that nurses should be deemed capable of undertaking the additional responsibilities that the new roles demanded. Some doctors reacted strongly to the issues of role expansion, which was difficult to understand, especially because these posts also provided recognition for some existing evolved roles in which entrepreneurial nurses were already delivering services comparable to elements of the Nurse Consultant role.

However, although some doctors initially opposed the development, many medical consultants proved to be enthusiastic supporters and were key in helping to design the new roles. Support has expanded and grown over time as medical consultants have continued to champion Nurse Consultant development, with the result that opposition to the role seems to have substantially diminished.

Nursing opposition

Some nurses, particularly those in specialist practitioner roles, were also strongly against the creation of Nurse Consultants. The view promulgated by many of these opponents was that this new role was unnecessary as specialist nurses were already undertaking the range of clinical roles proposed for Nurse Consultants. It is probable, however, that this opinion stemmed from the concern of specialist nurses that they, in their individual posts, might be displaced by new Nurse Consultants. This protectionism might have been fuelled by the guidance for making appointments to Nurse Consultant posts (NHS Executive, 1999a), which clearly advised that posts should not be designed around individuals and that recruitment should be subject to open competition. Although many specialist nurses were able to view the development of Nurse Consultant roles as an opportunity to be pursued, some expressed unease and, rather than seeing themselves as likely candidates for the potential Nurse Consultant posts, held the development to be a threat.

Quite clearly, however, the specialist nurse pool is the source from which many Nurse Consultants have been drawn, and as the role has become established, the career opportunity that the role affords specialist nurses has become more apparent. Nursing opposition to the role is now much less obvious, probably for this reason.

Opposition from managers

Some managers were also opposed to the development of the Nurse Consultant role, much of this opposition centring on the pay grade and cost of these posts. In 1999, the salary of nurse specialist practitioners varied from clinical grade F to grade I, the majority being graded at grade H. The new salary band for Nurse Consultants announced in 1999 was considerably higher than any other pre-existing nurse grade, its starting point being close to the maximum salary that a clinical nurse could earn at that time.

Managers voiced concern that the role would merely escalate the cost of nursing with little gain to clinical delivery, and some questioned the rationale of paying a price for clinical nursing that was considerably greater than that paid for a similar role, for example that of the specialist nurse practitioner. Some managers also disagreed with the principle that the complex and multifaceted nature of the Nurse Consultant role, combined with an increased level of clinical responsibility and accountability, demanded that the Nurse Consultant should be graded higher than other clinical nursing roles. These views probably influenced the way in which the salaries of proposed Nurse Consultant posts were determined by some managers.

Guidance relating to grading and the pay arrangements, as well as an assessment of the demands of the role, were set out in an *Advance Letter* (NHS Executive, 1999b), which also identified the factors to be considered when determining the appropriate starting point for the salary of each post. Although this guidance was available from the start of implementation, it does not seem to have created the desired level playing field for appointments. An early study of the establishment of Nurse Consultants (Guest et al, 2001) identified that although 68% of early Nurse Consultant posts were paid between £31,000 and £36,000, this hid considerable disparities in pay, the range being between £24,000 and £45,000.

Further fuel to managerial opposition was the fact that, traditionally, clinical nurses within the NHS were usually paid at a lower grade than middle and senior managers. The new pay scale for Nurse Consultants raised the prospect of a clinical nurse earning as much as, or even more than, a manager.

The view that Nurse Consultants were expensive was compounded by an additional factor. Department of Health guidance within HSC 1999/217 (NHS Executive, 1999a) recommended that each new post should be implemented with an identified job plan. This job plan was required to identify programmes for the 10 sessions of the working week, and although at least 50% of sessions were to be allocated to clinical practice, job plans were also to include dedicated sessions for teaching, research and administration. Therefore, in a week-by-week comparison, each Nurse Consultant post would provide fewer hours in direct clinical care than would an equivalent nurse specialist. Some managers focused on this narrow comparison to reach the conclusion that Nurse Consultants were poor value for money.

The managers who shared these views, and as a result opposed the development of the role, missed the point of one of the major drivers for the creation of the new role, i.e. to help to keep experienced and expert nurses in practice, rather than their having little choice but to leave clinical practice for jobs in management in order to achieve a higher income.

Opposition on the grounds of poor value for money has diminished over time as new innovative roles have been evaluated positively and Nurse Consultants have proved their value. What is not known, however, is whether or not opposition, which the pay differential issue generated, still exists and whether or not it continues to militate against the development of new posts.

By November 2000, a new strategy for the allied health professions heralded the extension of the Consultant role to Therapists, with the aim of:

- providing better outcomes for patients by improving quality and services
- providing a new career opportunity for experienced allied health professionals
- strengthening professional leadership.

Building on the Nurse Consultant initiative (DoH, 2000b), the strategy drew a clear distinction between 'Therapist Consultants' and Nurse Consultants. The strategy identified that each Therapist post would be structured around the same four core functions as those determined for Nurse Consultants:

- an expert practice function
- a professional leadership and consultancy function
- an education, training and development function
- a practice and service development, research and evaluation function.

This must be seen as an early clear endorsement by the Department of Health of its confidence in the value of Nurse Consultants.

What is apparent and not easy to link to any single factor is the uneven distribution of Nurse Consultant posts that can be seen across the NHS in England. It can be seen that there are some quite distinct differences in implementation between comparable organisations: in some, sizeable cohorts of Nurse Consultants have developed, yet in others perhaps a single post or sometimes even none exists.

Primary Care Trust (PCT) commissioners have adopted the development of the Nurse Consultant role with varying degrees of support. As commissioners of mental health, primary and secondary care services, PCTs must approve with the relevant provider any new developments or appointments that cannot be met from within the Trust's existing resources. With numerous competing demands on the financial resources of PCTs, the development of Nurse Consultant posts will depend upon the success of the business case to deliver on key priorities for the local health community.

Supportive environments

What should also be noted when considering the geography of the spread of Nurse Consultant posts is the possible impact of the presence or absence of a senior nursing figure in the locality who will champion such a new role. Clear differences in the number of posts proposed were seen during the early implementation period between those health authorities in which strong nurse leadership existed and those where nurse leadership had been marginalized.

Guest et al's (2001) preliminary evaluation of the establishment of Nurse Consultants identified that, during the introductory period, a lack of support from any senior manager or professional was a key problem for some Nurse Consultants, creating difficulties, anxiety and a sense of isolation. This was compounded by the fact that as Nurse Consultants were part of a new development, role models for the new post-holders were few and far between. This factor is likely to have become much less of an issue because, as the role has matured, pathfinder Nurse Consultants have themselves become excellent role models for mentoring newly appointed Nurse Consultants, thereby providing an excellent source of peer support.

There was concern generated from the nursing community regarding the potential loss of nurse leadership and its possible impact at the time when plans for foundation hospitals were announced in 2002. At that time, the composition of the board was, for all pre-existing hospital Trusts, required to include an Executive Director of Nursing, but the composition initially proposed for Foundation Trusts failed to require the inclusion of a nurse at director level. This omission generated considerable unease among nurses at the time because of the possible negative impact that this lack of senior nurse leadership could have on nursing development and innovation, not least on the development and support of the new Nurse Consultants. Intensive lobbying from nurse leaders took place to convince government ministers that the delivery of the government reform of the NHS, largely dependent on the work of nurses, would be affected if these nurse leaders did not have a designated place on the new boards. This lobbying was successful, bringing about a subsequent amendment to the Bill. All NHS Foundation Trust boards are now required to have a director who is a nurse or a midwife, thus securing nurse leadership at a senior and influential level of the NHS.

The reactions to the introduction of Nurse (and by extension Therapist) Consultants were mixed and varied. Reactions have been based upon a combination of role clarifying, role expectations, responsibilities and how these may influence and impact upon the working practices of other professions. As already outlined in detail in Chapters 2 and 3, it is essential, in order to avoid and redress these emerging issues, to set out parameters and boundaries early on. Furthermore, ensuring that NTCs are encouraged and empowered to undertake their role and responsibilities efficiently and effectively requires an organisational culture and working environment that is supportive and not restrictive. If these emerging issues associated with reactions and support are resolved, the impact of the NTC could be profound.

ESTABLISHING THE IMPACT OF THE NTC

Establishing the impact of the NTC is difficult, which is why an entire chapter is devoted to its evaluation. Some early measures of impact that could be considered are whether or not these posts complement or detract from promoting the Agenda for Change, qualifications on selection of the NTC and developing the role in the future.

Agenda for Change

The strategy to reform the pay structure for non-medical staff throughout the NHS, the *Agenda for Change* (DoH, 1999b), received approval for full-scale testing in June 2003, with early implementation in a number of sites. At the heart of the new pay system is a job evaluation scheme that aims to break down old-style demarcations with remuneration based on an assessment of responsibilities. Early indications are that Agenda for Change will have a positive impact on the development of the NTC role, not least because it will remove the clinical grading system, which was cited by *Making a Difference* (DoH, 1999a) as being a limitation on nursing reform and innovation.

Qualification for selection

A contentious point throughout the initial implementation phase has centred on the level of qualification deemed by those developing proposals for posts to be required of applicants for the Nurse Consultant role. Health circular guidance (NHSE, 1999a) quite clearly makes the point, throughout the document, that potential nurse, midwife and health visitor Consultants must be able to demonstrate considerable professional knowledge and skills, supported by participation in programmes of advanced learning, and that 'the nature of consultant posts will demand a portfolio of career-long learning, experience and formal education **usually** up to or beyond Master's degree level; research experience and a network of scholarship and publications **will** become the norm for appointments of this sort.'

Although eligibility does not, according to the guidance, depend on a requirement for a formal qualification, the elements of the role are quite clearly such that considerable learning and academic ability need to be demonstrated. The existence of formal qualification provides a simple and consistent assurance for recruitment selection panels. On the other hand, although a number of degree courses have existed for some time at both Bachelor's and Master's levels, only a relatively small number of postregistration nurses have been seconded and/or funded to undertake such qualifications by their employing organisations. However, Guest and Redfern (2001) found that the early group of appointees to Nurse Consultant posts possessed an impressive range of qualifications, 65% having either a PhD or a Master's level qualification, and a further 25% possessing a first degree. The implication is therefore that although the remaining 10% may have possessed other qualifications, a requirement for potential applicants to have possessed formal degree qualifications would have eliminated them from the application process. Appointment panels are still encouraged to consider the totality of a candidate's portfolio of experience and qualifications, along with evidence of professional competencies and a range of important personal attributes.

The pool of nurses from which potential Nurse Consultants were first drawn reflected the situation that existed in 1999 prior to the introduction of the new posts, but since the inception of Nurse Consultants, nurses have had the opportunity to consider the rationale for undertaking higher qualifications in preparation for future career opportunities, and this must now influence development pathways. The development of the Nurse Consultant role provides a clear incentive to nurses to develop clinical skills and remain clinically active while also pursuing supportive academic qualifications.

Development of the role

Initial applications to develop Nurse Consultant posts received during the first year resulted in the approval of a total of 451 posts nationally by November 2000 (DoH, 2000). The number of Nurse Consultants has since steadily increased until, by the end of 2003, the figure stood at just below 800. Key elements of *Making a Difference* (DoH, 1999a), particularly the Chief Nursing Officer's '10 key roles for nurses', were crucial in supporting and nurturing the development of an environment of innovation in nursing. What these did was support the development of an increasing level of autonomy for nurses, particularly related to prescribing medicines and ordering tests, alongside a reduction in restrictive practices.

Making a Difference has become a major enabler of the growth of roles and responsibilities of many nurses, especially those working at the frontline of the profession and particularly Nurse Consultants. Examples of the development of often innovative roles in nursing include Primary Medical Services pilots, NHS Direct, emergency care practitioners, etc. This is an important context for the development of the Nurse Consultant role because, without the associated developments and changes set out in *Making a Difference* and *The NHS Plan* (DoH, 2000b), the emancipation of nursing within which the role was to develop could never have been achieved.

The majority of early proposals for Nurse Consultants were developed within the secondary and tertiary care sectors. Increasingly, however, new posts are being developed and commissioned through partnership arrangements across health communities involving a range of clinicians, service managers, PCT commissioners, local universities and patient representatives.

In brief, as NTCs have begun to demonstrate their effectiveness in improving the patient experience by leading modernisation and service development, local health communities are beginning to establish NTC posts as a strategic approach to improve performance.

CONCLUSION: OPPORTUNITY FOR THE FUTURE

A range of drivers has emerged over recent times to indicate strongly that this developmental trend will continue. Of particular note is the change programme relating to the implications of a new contract for GPs (DoH, 2003a). The implications of the revised contract for General Medical Services, which was agreed in 2003, along with those changes related to the Choice initiative (DoH, 2003b), are extensive. The new roles and services that will need to develop so that the government's intention to offer patients greater choice and plurality of provision can be recognised as having an enormous potential for the roles of NTCs. Audited examples from innovative pilot schemes and international examples already exist to demonstrate the diverse roles that can be safely undertaken by nurses. Further evidence of the movement was found in the Chief Executive's Annual Report to the NHS (DoH, 2003c), which identified that the greatest growth in NHS activity for the year up to September 2003 was in new nurse-led services.

The Minister of State for Health, Dr John Reid, in a speech to nurse leaders at the annual Chief Nurses Conference in Brighton on 12 November 2003, was unequivocal in his view that nurses would be even more creative and developmental than ever before. He shared with the conference his vision for nursing, that 'nurses' talents need to be liberated and that it is the duty of those around them to support this change'. He urged the conference 'to be radical, to seize the gain and use the opportunity that nurses now have, to be everything they can be' (DoH, 2003d). This speech provided a clear indication of the government's view of nursing as a crucial enabler of modernisation of the NHS.

NTCs are at the forefront of innovative nursing and allied health practices, and the Department of Health is relying on nurses and the allied health professions, particularly NTCs, to take the initiative, creating and implementing new ideas. This movement can only be successful if nurse and allied health professional leaders focus their professional role on enabling and supporting innovation by providing a safety net of knowledge, information and visible support for nurse/therapist entrepreneurs in order to minimise the risk to which they may be exposed. This leadership role is a key role that nurse/allied health professional leaders, particularly leads/directors, must fulfil, otherwise the progress of nursing innovation will be hampered in its growth.

One of the factors leading to the successful establishment of NTC posts has been the ability of those developing them to articulate the role as a solution to a local problem with service delivery. For example, the first statements about Nurse Consultants identified the importance of these roles in leading change, often across disciplines and organisational boundaries. This element of clinical and service change clearly differentiated the role of the Nurse Consultant from that of the specialist nurse. The former can be described as having a unique role in terms of its impact on the modernisation of services, far beyond the functioning of a narrow clinical speciality. An example of this would be the impact of a Nurse Consultant in intermediate care on the development of care outside the acute sector and on the establishment of new pathways of care that lead to new, primary models of care with appropriate specialist clinical support. Thus, in developing proposals for NTCs, it has been important to move beyond the desire to provide career opportunities for nursing/allied health professional staff with specific clinical interests to the development of roles that meet pressing needs within health and social care communities to modernise the way in which services are delivered.

SUMMARY OF KEY POINTS

- To provide an executive and managerial perceptive of the NTC, it is imperative to outline in sequence the events associated with the evolution of the post.
- The journey from policy to reality has proved to be eventful, particularly for the early pioneers of the NTC role.
- The development of NTCs depends on the unswerving support, enthusiasm and persuasive powers of key nurse, therapist, medical and managerial leaders.

- Reactions to the introduction of the NTCs were mixed and varied. They were based upon a combination of role clarifying, role expectations, responsibilities and how these might influence and impact upon the working practices of other professions.
- Early impact measures that could be considered are whether or not these posts complement or detract from promoting the *Agenda for Change* (DoH, 1999b), qualifications on selection of the NTC and developing the role in the future.
- NTCs are at the forefront of innovative nursing and allied health practices, and the Department of Health is relying on nurses and the allied health professions, particularly NTCs, to take the initiative, creating and implementing new ideas.

RECOMMENDED READING

Department of Health (1998) Nurse Consultants (1). Health Service Circular 1998/161. DoH, London.
NHS Executive (2000) *Meeting the Challenge: A Strategy for the Allied Health Professions*. DoH, London.

REFERENCES

Department of Health (1998a) *Nurse Consultants*. Health Service Circular 1998/161. DoH, London.
Department of Health (1998b) *A Consultation on a Strategy for Nursing Midwifery and Health Visiting*. Health Service Circular 1998/04. DoH, London.
Department of Health (1999a) *Making a Difference: Strengthening the Nursing, Midwifery and Health Visiting Contribution to Health and Healthcare*. DoH, London.
Department of Health (1999b) *Agenda for Change – Modernising the NHS Pay System*. HSC 199/227. DoH, London.
Department of Health (2000a) Press release 2000/0690. DoH, London.
Department of Health (2000b) The NHS Plan: a plan for investment, a plan for reform. DoH, London.
Department of Health (2003a) *New GMS Contract and Changes to GP Premises Funding Arrangements*. DoH, London.
Department of Health (2003b) *Choice of Hospitals Guidance for PCTs, NHS Trusts and SHAs on Offering Patients Choice of Where They Are Treated*. DoH, London.
Department of Health (2003c) *Chief Executive's Report to the NHS*. DoH, London.
Department of Health (2003d) Press release 2003/0462. DoH, London.
Guest D, Redfern S (2001) *A Preliminary Evaluation of the Establishment of Nurse Midwife and Health Visitor Consultants*. King's College, London.
NHS Executive (1999a) *Nurse Midwife and Health Visitor Consultants. Establishing Posts and Making Appointments*. HSC 1999/217. NHSE.
NHS Executive (1999b) *Nurse, Midwife and Health Visitor Consultants 1999/2000. Advance letter* (NM) 2/1999. NHSE.
NHS Executive (2000) *Meeting the Challenge: A Strategy for the Allied Health Professions*. DoH, London.

8 SUPPORTING THE NURSE/THERAPIST CONSULTANT

Rob McSherry, Wendy Francis, John Campbell, Tim Renshaw and Margaret Murray

INTRODUCTION

This chapter outlines the importance of developing ways of obtaining support to help with implementing and evaluating the Nurse/Therapist Consultant (NTC) post. Practical advice and guidance for obtaining internal and/or external support through networking, partnerships building are detailed.

According to previous writers, the roles and responsibilities of the NTC can be seen to be wide ranging and varied, a view confirmed by Harker (2001) and Coady (2003). This suggests that each NTC will need a supportive framework in place in order to carry out the role successfully.

WHAT CONSTITUTES SUPPORT, AND WHY IT IS IMPORTANT TO THE NTC

Much of the emerging literature and evaluative studies of the NTC role emphasise support as a fundamental part of the post (Guest et al, 2001). The Chambers Dictionary (1990) defines support as 'to sustain, to maintain, to strengthen, to uphold, to back up, to nourish and to strengthen'. From this, we see that support is not just associated with physical structures, but the meaning in this context is one of emotional support, which must be embedded within the organisation for the benefit of staff members and patients.

Support is important when encouraging staff to apply for these new posts. Craik and McKay (2003) state:

> *Crucial to the creation of consultant therapists is the need for occupational therapy managers to support and mentor the development of sufficient numbers of therapists with the potential to become consultant therapists.*

Once in post, Guest et al (2001) point out that a:

> *key problem for some consultants was a lack of support from any senior managers or professionals; while some had very positive stories to tell, others said that the role sponsor had abandoned any subsequent responsibility.*

In order for the NTC to realise the potential of the post, four key elements of support need to be present: physical, psychological, social and support staff. With these present, NTCs can develop their practice and start to realise the potential of the role. They will then be able to develop a supportive environment and provide support to others within the workplace, enabling NTCs to develop a supportive

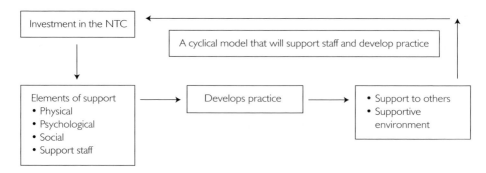

Figure 8.1   A cyclical model that will support staff and develop best practice led by the NTC

and sustaining environment. One practical measure that could be implemented is the setting up of 'buddy systems' or a 'critical companion', from which ideas and issues can be shared and discussed in a non-threatening way with a colleague.

Activity 8.1   *Reflective question*

Ways of supporting the NTC

Note down types of support and ways of supporting the NTC.

Read on and compare your findings with those in the Activity Feedback at the end of this section.

Physical support

Office space and desktop workstations are in short supply in many institutions, but it is vital that an area is available in which NTCs can perform their various non-clinical or administrative duties. Access to information technology and Internet facilities is essential in modern health care. The use of a PC with a range of software packages that includes an email account should be in place from the outset. A portable PC or a facility to pick messages up from distant locations together with other communication systems, for example a mobile telephone and/or long-range pager, will help as individuals will find themselves in many different locations as their role evolves.

Resources

Resources can include office space and information technology, but for most NTCs it is about having sufficient administrative support to assist them in developing, implementing and evaluating their role. Each post that is proposed includes a bid for secretarial support for up to a 0.5 whole-time equivalent appointment. Whether this secretarial support is to be allocated from an individual who is already in post or identified as a new appointment should be addressed so that it can be co-ordinated appropriately. It may be difficult at the beginning of the NTC role to identify the full range of duties that the secretary will cover, but as the role develops and more responsibilities are identified for the NTC, this support becomes more important.

Linked with resources is the notion of 'dress code'. Some NTC posts will have a clear clinical focus that requires a uniform or specialist clothing. Again, this should be identified prior to commencement. Decisions on uniform must address the dilemma of creating a role that is identifiable to the public and the team while simultaneously establishing a role that is integral to the team. Those NTCs who choose to wear smart professional attire rather than uniform must consider how they will be differentiated by the public from the mass of other hospital staff in similar clothing.

There will undoubtedly be a resource implication and requirement for ongoing training and personal professional development for all those appointed to the NTC role. Whether these sessions take the form of university modules and courses, study days, network meetings, clinical updates or support groups, a cost will be incurred for attendance and travelling. The appraisal process should help appointees to identify priorities for training, but the application process and the budget allocation should be transparent. It is imperative for the NTC to have sufficient support and the resources to function efficiently and effectively.

Psychological and social support

Psychological and social support systems are essential for ensuring that NTCs have an appropriate place to share ideas, express concerns and seek clarification. This must be within an open supportive climate and non-threatening working environment. Psychological and social support could be obtained through peer/individual clinical supervision (outlined later in the chapter) or by organising regular formal debriefing sessions.

In summary, many of the issues that relate to support are inherent within the organisation. Failing to put a supportive infrastructure in place risks isolating the NTC and will lessen the relevance of the post.

TAKING THE NTC FORWARD: DEVELOPING A SUPPORTIVE FRAMEWORK

Reid and Metcalfe (2001) believe that a major step forward lies in the job description being clear, ensuring that the applicant, employer and team members have a firm understanding of the role.

Perceptions, assumptions and meanings of the role will undoubtedly be influenced by organisational cultures, values and beliefs (Manley, 2001).

A framework for seeking out and obtaining support can be outlined as follows:

- As identified in Chapters 2 and 3, seek out and clarify the scope, remit and parameters of the post with your employer, colleagues, peers and users.
- Critically review your job descriptions and contract of employment, and highlight key priorities so that an operational/performance strategy and action

plan can be developed around the support that you may require. Identify who could provide this so you can achieve your aims and objectives.

- Set up interviews and meetings with employers, colleagues, peers and users, as well as other NTCs, to seek their opinions and share and clarify ideas relating to the post.
- Do not be afraid to seek out sources of help and support.
- Once the 'fact-finding' is complete, i.e. you have gathered enough information about the post, identify key systems, departments or individual(s) who may be able to offer support in advancing and evaluating the role.
- Link support to your *own* continued professional development (CPD), individual personal review and personal and professional development plan (McSherry and Bassett, 2002).

Building internal and external support systems

Professionals working in health and social care are familiar with the process of reflection and clinical supervision as part of self-development, providing insight into factors that drive individuals and influence practice development by altering service provision (McSherry and Bassett, 2002). An expansion of roles in health and social care has been linked to the importance of providing support organisationally, professionally and personally to the individual. More successful developments have had such values underpinning the process (Benner, 1984). If this support is pivotal to the success of service and role development, it is, by implication, crucial in the development of the NTC role. The difficulties and challenges facing some NTCs lie in identifying the internal and external support available to them (Box 8.1).

Box 8.1   Ways of building supportive frameworks and being supportive

Internal to the organisation	External to the organisation
• Executive, senior management and team meetings	• Professional and voluntary groups
• Journal clubs or reflective groups	• Conferences: locally, regionally, nationally or internationally
• Professional forums	• Professional support groups and networks
• Networks	• Mentorship
• Mentorship, buddy system	• CPD and staff development
• CPD and staff development	

NB: This list is not exhaustive.

It is evident from Box 8.1 that sources of internal and external support are in fact available for NTCs. MacPhee (2002) stated that NTCs 'must understand the nature of support networks to improve patient care, staff satisfaction, and retention'. Support networks or groups must provide a balance between social, functional and psychological support so that NTCs can develop best practice. New NTCs should take time to invest in building a supportive network using a variety and diverse range of internal and external sources such as those identified in Figure 8.1 and Box 8.1.

A supportive network should be developed for the following reasons:

- to ensure that you have the help and support of colleagues
- to share ideas
- to build a supportive personal and professional network
- to develop professional networks to share developments in practice
- to encourage and engage staff so that they become acquainted and familiar with your position, role and responsibilities
- to develop strategies to deal with work-related stress and enhance self-esteem, efficacy and control.

The support structures that have developed vary in their format, and others have evolved with the extension of NTC posts themselves. This is not surprising when you consider that one of the core competencies of these posts is leadership. NTCs have not waited for support to arrive but, where support has been limited, have sought out more formal support networks and other methods to help their development and needs. But why is networking so important?

Networking and partnership development

Support networks have a local, regional or national component (Table 8.1), some being more successful than others with a different organisational infrastructure.

Table 8.1   NTC networks

Network	Organisation	Web address
Consultant Nurse Network	Royal College of Nursing and Foundation of Nursing Studies	http://fons.org/networks/cnn/index.htm
Link in Nurse Consultant Site (LINC)	University of Northumbria, Royal College of Nursing and NHS Direct, South East Region, Hampshire	http://online.unn.ac.uk/faculties/hswe/research/PDRP/LinkNurse.htm

It is good to see from Table 8.1 that joint working, collaboration and partnership-building between and across organisations and regions in the United Kingdom are developing useful and practical ways to support the NTC. Although the networks are primarily orientated towards Nurse Consultants, it is strongly recommended that these evolve to encompass Therapist Consultants as well. The scope and purpose of these networks and groups should be relevant to *all* NTCs.

Nationally, the Consultant Nurse Network, a joint venture between the Royal College of Nursing and the Foundation of Nursing Studies, aims 'to provide a UK-wide forum for consultant nurses to share ideas and learning. To provide opportunities for mutual challenge, support and to influence policy' (Consultant

Nurse Network, 2003). Similarly, the Link in Nurse Consultant site (LINC) was established by leads in practice development from across the country aiming to 'provide an opportunity for nurse consultants to communicate and develop practice knowledge without the necessity of planning time out of the diary to attend meetings or conferences' (LINC, 2002).

Regionally, we have witnessed the establishment and launch of the South Yorkshire Nurse Consultant Group (University of Sheffield, 2003), with a remit for sharing and pooling knowledge, skills and expertise in order to improve patient care within the local context. The Northern Region was one area that provided a focus for this, and within five months of the first posts being established, the North East and Yorkshire Regional Health Authority had facilitated a regional meeting attended by all Nurse Consultants in post at that time (September 2000). Such meetings created a support network within which individual Consultants could meet and share practical elements of their role development, as well as accessing current information on relevant issues. Meetings were held quarterly until the regional health authorities were disbanded. Since then, arrangements have been made for running a similar format within the Strategic Health Authority. The Leadership Centre has initiated a group for allied health professional (AHP) Consultants, which has met monthly in London to provide support and guidance to the small number of Consultants currently in post.

As more posts develop nationally, with particular reference to similar areas of clinical practice, national meetings have been held, providing an opportunity for some NTCs to discuss developments in the context of the national agenda. These meetings have been co-ordinated by the Department of Health in such areas as tissue viability, public health, emergency care and cardiac care. The Royal College of Midwives provides a network for Midwife Consultants. The informal network and contact that is maintained between formal meetings is helpful for continued professional growth.

NTCs developing support in this way have demonstrated that this concept is critical for their successful role development, and that the time and resources have been well invested, having a positive impact. This echoes the work of Manley (2000) when she discusses the empowerment of staff and cites Rodwell (1996) and Gibson (1991), who identify that staff can not be empowered but must work to empower themselves; the staff involved in such roles will tend to challenge themselves (Manley, 2001). Demonstrating this behaviour and having a culture in which it is safe to challenge and, by critically evaluating alternatives, all service provision to expand means that it is possible to respond creatively to patients' needs. In the context of role expansion, it was for this very reason that the Nurse/AHP Consultant roles were developed. They were created to work across boundaries and deliver new ways of working, providing leadership and demonstrating the value of new ways of working with the patient as the focus of the agenda.

Staff applying for NTC posts are, by the nature of the person and the job specifications, senior staff with a wide body of previous experience that has provided them with a personal support network. Some people find this in family or friends, colleagues or individuals within their current organisation. The value of this resource needs to be acknowledged, as this support network will help the new NTC who has to deal with feelings of isolation and confusion.

The limitations of these emerging support networks or groups are minimal given the fact that any network or group that encourages the sharing and spreading of practice could be seen to be positive. The difficulties faced by some NTCs lies in accessing and freeing up the time to participate. The option to join support networks and groups is usually voluntary, creating the need for networks and groups to have clear and specific terms of reference, aims, purpose and vision so that members can identify the potential gains from joining them. Throughout this book, time management emerges as a key factor in the day-to-day work of the NTC. The participation in or attendance at support networks or groups must be justified through documented role, organisational and/or personal/professional development.

Support networks or groups may in future become difficult to manage and organise as the number of NTCs rises. This may be because the increasing number of NTCs challenges the support network's potential terms of reference, aims and/or purpose as a result of issues associated with representation, generality or indeed speciality. Perhaps support networks should be tailored to specific specialities or professionals, although this could be viewed as a contradiction to promoting partnership-building, collaborating and modernisation. The emergence of several different support groups widens choice and creates competition but has the potential to affect the group's viability and sustainability, depending on the number joining. There are usually no costs or fees to join support networks or groups, depending upon the sources of funding. However, although the cost of joining such groups is minimal, there will be a hidden cost in terms of the time taken to attend. The development of Internet support networks or telephone conferencing/master classes could resolve these issues.

In summary, internal and external support networks or groups have a major role to play in encouraging and engaging NTCs to share and spread advances and evaluations in their practice. The potential benefits from such networks or groups are enormous, outweighing many of the limitations. Having explored the strengths and limitations of networks and groups, the next section depicts two key ways of supporting the NTC role: action learning and learning sets, and clinical supervision.

ACTION LEARNING AND LEARNING SETS

This section has been adapted from McSherry and Bassett (2002), with permission. Over the past decade, action learning has become a popular method of promoting personal and professional growth, sharing and learning from experiences (past and present), yet its effect on patient outcomes has been limited. In spite of the this, action learning continues to be utilised in business and management, education, and health and social care service and academic organisations to promote change. The popularity and usefulness of action learning as a method for learning originate from its definition (Revans, 1979):

> *a means of development, intellectual, emotional or physical, that requires its subjects, through responsible involvement in some real, complex and stressful problems, to achieve intended change sufficient to improve his observable behaviours henceforth in the problem field.*

Action learning in this instance supports the development of the NTC because the posts are new, challenging, stressful and rewarding but fundamentally important to the modernisation of services and the professions. Action learning, if used effectively, has the potential to provide emotional support and intellectual challenge through shared learning; personal and professional growth; the creation of a mechanism for the iterative exploration of alternative action in the light of new insights; and change. Action learning used for this purpose provides a 'continuous process of learning and reflection, supported by colleagues, with the intention of getting things done' (McGill and Beaty, 1995). Action learning in this context is ideal for the NTC because it focuses on bringing individuals together in small groups, known as 'learning sets', in which members' ideas can be challenged in a supportive, non-threatening environment with the support and guidance of a set facilitator. The learning set provides a balance of emotional and intellectual challenge 'through comradeship and insightful questioning which enables each member to act and learn effectively on three levels' (Bird, 2002): first to *present* the problem to be tackled, second to *explore* what is being learned about oneself, and third to consider the *process* of learning itself. These principles of action learning complement the NTC because the role is primarily about presenting, exploring and responding to challenge and change. What better way is there to achieve the latter than to share and work with individuals in a similar plight? In our experiences with action learning to date, action learning sets form a unique type of learning community or cohort because members come together in a voluntary and supportive way and form a contract to share, help and learn with and from each other.

Action learning is different from traditional ways of teaching and learning, and is ideal for advancing and evaluating the NTC role because it focuses on the individual's current, rather than past, experience and situation, which requires active involvement in resolving real, not historic, case studies (Figure 8.2).

According to Figure 8.2, action learning is an ideal way in which to promote and support NTCs because they can become a set member, which can enable them to discuss ideas/issues associated with their role and responsibilities and be supported in a structured way to advance their practice. Likewise, it enables them to undertake training to become a facilitator of action learning. From our personal experience, it would complement the development, implementation and evaluation aspects of the NTC role because it is an ideal way of:

- advancing practice within a team and organisation
- encouraging and assuring effective collaboration and communication

- providing support in an informal, non-threatening, structured way
- networking
- sharing and disseminating practice.

Traditional Learning	Action learning
Historic case studies	Current case studies
Individual orientation	Group-based learning
Learning about others	Learning about self and others
Studying other organisations	Studying own organisation
Programme knowledge	Questions plus programmed knowledge
Planning	Planning and doing
Arm's Length	Arm in arm with clients
Input based	Output/result based
Past oriented	Present and future oriented
Low risk	Higher risk
Passive	Active

Figure 8.2   (Adapted from McSherry and Bassett, 2002)

The advantages of action learning to health and social care and those professionals with or without a remit for advancing and evaluating practice or practice development can be categorised into several benefits:

- the process empowers the participants by encouraging them to take charge of their own problems/issues
- it encourages problem-solving skills
- it accommodates a wide variety of situations because of its flexibility in design
- transfer of learning is increased.

If NTCs engage in and apply action learning to support their own and colleagues' learning, the potential benefits to their role, organisation and patients are profound, on several accounts. The processes are engaging, encouraging, empowering and, most importantly, evolving, arguably the essence of effective clinical and transformational leadership.

The challenge to action learning lies in demonstrating its actual value to individuals, team or organisational performances because of the flexibility of its method and diversity in accommodating the uniqueness of each learning set and its participants. Although it remains difficult to measure and quantify action learning, from our experiences of using it within health and social care practice and education, the impact on individual personal learning and development is vast. The difficulty for some NTCs, like other health and social care professionals and organisations, is in sharing and disseminating experiences at a local, regional or international level.

In short, action learning has an important part to play in advancing and evaluating the NTC role in the future. Action learning provides an important set of principles and processes for sharing and spreading ideas and initiatives in a non-threatening, supportive environment, for both NTCs and staff. Engaging in action learning is paramount. Likewise, becoming a facilitator of action learning could become your ally. Having explored the potential advantages and limitations of action learning to the NTC, what about clinical supervision?

ESTABLISHING A SUPPORTIVE FRAMEWORK THROUGH CLINICAL SUPERVISION

This section is adapted from McSherry and Bassett (2002) with permission. Clinical supervision is defined as 'a formal arrangement that enables nurses, midwives and health visitors to discuss their work regularly with another experienced professional. Clinical supervision involves reflecting on practice in order to learn from experience and improve confidence' (Kohner, 1994). Clinical supervision is described as a formal process of professional support and learning, enabling individual practitioners to develop knowledge and competence, assume responsibility for their own practice and enhance consumer protection and safety of care in complex situations. It is central to the process of learning and the scope of professional practice, and should be seen as a means of encouraging self-assessment and analytical and reflective skills (DoH, 1993). Having reflected upon the above definitions and descriptions of clinical supervision, it is easy to see why it has the potential to support NTCs. Our rationale for this is because the core principles behind clinical supervision focus on (Kohner, 1994):

- safeguarding standards
- promoting professional development and expertise
- delivering and evaluating the quality care.

The above are arguably all key elements within the role, scope and parameters of the NTC. The challenge for individuals, teams and organisations is in utilising a model(s) of clinical supervision to become an informal yet supportive framework for advancing or evaluating practice. Bassett (1999) provides an excellent guide to implementing clinical supervision, accounting for the practicalities and challenges by drawing upon a variety of experts from within the clinical and practice development setting. The text provides an opportunistic framework for implementing and evaluating practice, along with an outline of the advantages and disadvantages of using such a method of providing support for individuals, teams or an organisation.

One such clinical supervision group was a rich source of support. The six members worked geographically close to each other but came from two local Acute Trusts and one Community Trust, with a wealth of previous experience and varied clinical practice. As with all clinical supervision, the individual problems were discussed in the safety and collaboration of the group, generating solutions to problems or providing empathy even if a solution to the problem was unavailable. When discussing clinical supervision, Goodyear (1997) suggests that this increased self-awareness contributes to the standards of care with professional collaboration, enhancing the value of such contribution from individuals; this was demonstrated within the dynamics of this group. Case study 8.1 below details the systems and processes involved in setting up group supervision.

NOT GOING IT ALONE

In brief, the chapter reinforces the need for NTCs to develop support frameworks, networks or groups in order to advance and evaluate the role, personal and professional growth, mechanisms for sharing and spreading ideas. What emerges from this chapter is that there is no need to 'go it alone' or indeed to feel isolated because the support, help and guidance is out there. It is all a question of seeking out and finding what best suits your needs and unique position. Remember that support can come from internal or external to the organisation.

Activity 8.1 *Feedback*

Ways of supporting the NTC

There are many different ways of ensuring that NTCs are supported to undertake their role efficiently and effectively; peer support, networking and action learning have been discussed here. Support needs to be physical, structural, functional and psychological, and should be regarded as an inherent part of the package before the post begins.

CONCLUSION

Support is crucial to advancing and evaluating the NTC role. Support needs to be planned, structured and varied depending on the uniqueness of the post and organisational environment. Ensuring that the NTC is supported is a joint responsibility between individual and employer. Support could be internal and/or external, within or away from the organisation, but more importantly it should complement and support both the NTC in the role and the individual's personal and professional growth.

SUMMARY OF KEY POINTS

- In order to accommodate the diversity of the roles and responsibilities of the post, a flexible set of mechanisms need to be put in place to support the NTC.
- The word 'support' means different things to different people depending upon the place, context and situation.
- The emerging literature and evaluation studies on the role of the NTC highlight support as a fundamental element in the success of the post.

- Four primary elements emerge as being crucial to achieving a holistic framework for support: physical, resource related, psychological and supportive/supporter.
- Action learning, if used effectively, has the potential to provide emotional support and intellectual challenge to provide new insights and change practice.
- The challenge for individuals, teams and organisations lies in utilising a model(s) of clinical supervision to develop an informal but supportive framework for advancing or evaluating practice.

CASE STUDY 8.1	CLINICAL SUPERVISION: PRACTICAL EXPERIENCE OF IMPLEMENTING GROUP CLINICAL SUPERVISION WITH NURSE CONSULTANTS

Wendy Francis

Setting the context

Clinical supervision is not a new concept. It has occurred informally within nursing for many years, but it has only recently been understood and acknowledged that clinical supervision informs the clinical governance agenda (McSherry et al, 2002). To promote evidence for clinical governance, the Commission for Health Inspection and Audit, and audit and professional development programmes, clinical supervision now requires a robust framework.

Within the framework of clinical governance, nurses and health visitors have developed a strong quality orientation, focusing on standards development, monitoring and audit methodologies, and increasingly on evidence-based practice. Their practice has been guided by professional self-regulation supported by clinical supervision (DoH, 1999). It was recognised early on that the first and second groups of NTCs appeared to be clinically isolated. Although there were regional meetings, held on a 3-monthly basis, these meetings did not allow an intensive exploration of the implications of these new roles. It soon became evident there was need for an environment that would support and challenge our clinical practice, especially as we were the first NTCs in the area. I had previously implemented clinical supervision across a Trust and suggested the idea of formulating a similar process and structure for these first six NTCs.

Various authors (Butterworth and Faugier, 1992; United Kingdom Central Council (UKCC), 1996; Bond and Holland, 1998; Royal College of Nursing, 2000) exemplified the process of clinical supervision, and although the UKCC (now known as the Nursing and Midwifery Council) at the time recommended and published a document on clinical supervision, it did not state that it was a requirement of re-registration. The UKCC position statement (1996) included six key statements (Box 8. 2).

Box 8.2   The UKCC's key statements on clinical supervision

Key Statement One
Clinical supervision supports practice, enabling practitioner to *maintain and promote standards of care*.

Key Statement Two
Clinical supervision is a *practice-focused, professional relationship* involving a practitioner reflecting on practice by a skilled supervisor.

Key Statement Three
The *process* of clinical supervision should be developed by practitioners and managers according to local circumstances. Ground rules should be agreed so that practitioners and supervisors approach clinical supervision openly, confidently and are aware of what is involved.

Key Statement Four
Every practitioner should have *access* to clinical supervision. Each supervisor should supervise a realistic number of practitioners.

Key Statement Five
Preparation for supervisors can be effected using 'in house' or external education programmes. The principle and relevance of clinical supervision should be included in pre and post-registration education programmes.

Key Statement Six
Evaluation of clinical supervision is needed to assess how it influences care; practice, standards and the service evaluation systems should be determined locally.

Activity 8.2   *Reflective question*

The benefits of introducing clinical supervision, and how to adapt the process to your clinical area

As you read this section, think about your own clinical area with the following in mind. Note down the possible benefits of introducing clinical supervision and how you could adapt the process to suit your clinical area.

Read on and compare your findings with those in the Activity Feedback at the end of this section.

The beginnings

Clinical supervision cannot be taken lightly, and it requires a skilled supervisor to provide one-to-one supervision. We suggested that we had group supervision, which required a different set of skills.

We agreed at our first meeting that we wanted to implement group clinical supervision sessions. There were many elements of clinical supervision that we needed to debate, and this laid down the foundations for the future clinical supervision sessions. In fact, the process of creating a safe environment had unknowingly commenced. Bond and Holland (1998) describe different modes of supervision such as pairs, triads and group supervision. We decided we would opt for the group mode. Within group supervision there are, however, different ways to conduct the supervision session. According to Bond and Holland (1998), it could be one of the following:

- peer colleagues within the same discipline, led by a supervisor who was either more experienced in the same field or had a specialist interest
- a group with peer colleagues and mixed disciplines led by a supervisor with group facilitation skills
- group with peer colleagues of the same discipline that was led by each group member in turn
- a peer group of colleagues from a variety of disciplines, led by group members in turn.

Having reflected upon the work of Bond and Holland (1998), we decided to opt for the last method as we felt this was most appropriate to our needs. Although we were all nurses, a range of specialisms was represented, including public health, spinal assessment, palliative and cancer care, forensic psychiatry, intermediate care and emergency care.

After choosing the mode of group peer supervision, the next decision was whether or not to have an external facilitator. There was the possibility of having an independent consultant who was familiar with group clinical supervision, for example one from a counselling or psychology background. The other options open to us were to involve someone from the wider region or another NTC colleague who was not part of our group.

What factors influenced our decision?

For group supervision, a facilitator or supervisor requires certain skills and experiences to provide an environment that will ensure effective supervision. It goes without saying that all supervisors should adhere to the core characteristics of a helping relationship identified by Rogers (1952). They will not only require the individual skills identified in Figure 8.3, but also be able to use them at different times throughout supervision depending on the specific interaction taking place. It would be the supervisor's role, through close observation and intuition, to make an assessment of the appropriate skill/s required at that moment. The most essential elements to possess for group supervision are skills in group dynamics, facilitation and empowerment.

By the time an individual is appointed to the position of NTC, it is acknowledged and assumed that they will, because of the seniority of the role, have already demonstrated many skills, competencies and expertise, and possess certain attributes. Within the NTCs in the group, we had approximately 100 years of National Health Service nursing experience, which, we agreed, meant that we had the abilities and enough skills to be able to utilise a group approach to clinical supervision.

Hawkins and Shohet (1989) have described the advantages and disadvantages of peer facilitation in groups; we agreed that there were more advantages to us as a group of newly appointed NTCs to rotate the facilitation within our group.

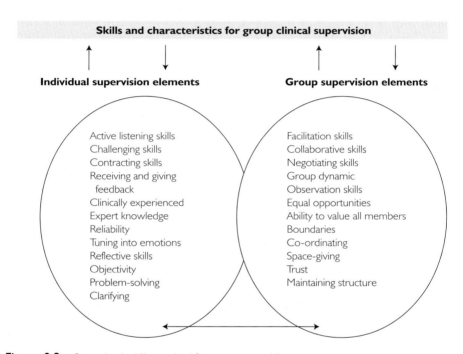

Skills and characteristics for group clinical supervision

Individual supervision elements

Active listening skills
Challenging skills
Contracting skills
Receiving and giving
  feedback
Clinically experienced
Expert knowledge
Reliability
Tuning into emotions
Reflective skills
Objectivity
Problem-solving
Clarifying

Group supervision elements

Facilitation skills
Collaborative skills
Negotiating skills
Group dynamic
Observation skills
Equal opportunities
Ability to value all members
Boundaries
Co-ordinating
Space-giving
Trust
Maintaining structure

Figure 8.3 Supervisor's skills required for group supervision

Setting the contract

For a peer group to be effective, it is essential to formulate a contract. Clear boundaries of confidentiality and the accountability of each of the participants in the group need to be discussed during the first meeting. Hawkins and Shohet (1989) stated that a contract of ground rules should be negotiated at the start of any supervisory relationship to protect both the person giving and the person receiving supervision. Another reason for formulating a contract is to have clear, agreed processes, should issues arise, that can be openly addressed because this is part of the contract and the group have made a commitment to each member. For example, if it is agreed that the group meet every month at a designated time but members are not attending or are continually leaving early, the group can safely raise this issue under the commitment that members made to each other when formulating the contract. More sensitive issues such as confidentiality can also be raised through this approach.

It was therefore agreed to set a contract between all the NTCs, and we spent the first session deciding what was important to enable us to feel safe to share. The contract in Box 8.3 was agreed.

Box 8.3   Clinical supervision contract

CONTRACT
Group clinical supervision for NTCs

AIMS OF THE GROUP
Clinical Supervision is to provide a safe environment for us to:-

- support each other
- critically reflect on current practice
- develop beyond the traditional nursing boundaries and develop professional practice
- share our experiences as NTCs
- investigate problematic areas of our roles
- explore the more risky elements of our role.

CONFIDENTIALITY
The group clinical supervision session is confidential between all members of the group.
Confidentiality will be maintained except in cases where professional conduct issues arise. These must be dealt with in accordance with professional guidelines, with the knowledge of both or all parties involved.
If these issues arise, they will be discussed within the group and a formalised action plan will be formulated to deal with the issue.

Time: – To meet for two hours every two months; to be reviewed every six months

Venue: – To be rotated at different locations.

Record-keeping: – To complete the records at each session. The documentation to be agreed and signed by all present at that session (see record-keeping form below).

A nominated group member to take responsibility for holding these and bringing them to each session. If he or she is unable to attend the required documentation to be given to another group member.

Supervisor: – The supervisor facilitation role will rotate. This will be discussed at the beginning of each session to determine who will take on that role for the session.

Attendance: – We will endeavour to attend every session. If unable to attend apologies to be sent to another member of the group.

Expectations

- statements are owned and group members speak from their own experience
- members show unconditional positive regard
- members are to be open and honest
- to commit to each member to attend where possible
- to review the process and model of supervision before six months if they are not working

Name: _____ Signature: _____ Date: _____

Name: _____ Signature: _____ Date: _____

Name: _____ Signature: _____ Date: _____

Name: _____ Signature: _____ Date: _____

Name: _____ Signature: _____ Date: _____

Name: _____ Signature: _____ Date: _____

PEER GROUP CLINICAL SUPERVISION NTC RECORD LOG

Date: _____

Key areas of discussion: _____

_____

_____

_____

Agreed action (if applicable): _____

_____

_____

_____

_____

Next supervision appointment: _____

Facilitator: _____   _____   _____

          (Print)   (Signature)   (Date)

Supervisee: _____   _____   _____

          (Print)   (Signature)   (Date)

Supervisee:			
	(Print)	(Signature)	(Date)
Supervisee:			
	(Print)	(Signature)	(Date)
Supervisee:			
	(Print)	(Signature)	(Date)
Supervisee:			
	(Print)	(Signature)	(Date)

Structure of the clinical supervision sessions

When a group of nurses meet, it is inevitable that 'informal networking' will take place. It is, however, critical that this catching-up and chatting does not, even though it is absolutely relevant, become clinical supervision. This point is highlighted because many supervision groups have reported that they only chat or complain, and some of the group members question the need to go to supervision. If a group develops in this way, this is not clinical supervision. Even more importantly, when we consider the constraints on professionals' time, is it crucial that supervision is structured and the sessions have a purpose.

The structure of the session was divided into welcome, setting the agenda, discussion and completing.

Welcome (10 minutes)

Recognising that the NTCs required networking time, we built into the structure of the session a **welcoming** time, which included making refreshments and networking.

Setting the agenda (10 minutes)

During this time, we agreed the facilitator for the session, followed up on issues raised at the last session and asked members who would like some discussion time. At this point, we usually also asked how much time people needed and sometimes negotiated how much time could be allotted to an individual person, especially if several wished to speak.

Discussion (1 hour 30 minutes, with a 10 minute refreshment break)

Case discussion, clinical experiences and issues were discussed in detail. During this time, the facilitator's role was to ensure that the person bringing the topic received the agreed time and space to explain and explore the issue. It was crucial that the facilitator took on the time-keeping and encouraged a fair discussion among the group, using the appropriate skills identified in figure 8.3.

Completing (10 minutes)

This section can sometimes be rushed due to inappropriate timing so it must be emphasised that this is part of the process and not an afterthought. Within this section, the facilitator clarified and summarised the issues raised, as well as any actions that needed to be addressed and by whom. The record-keeping for the session was also completed, within this time. See record log.

Clinical supervision themes

Here are some of the themes that have emerged from the supervision group over a period of two years. These are emerging themes and reflect the general opinion of other NTCs across the United Kingdom. The issues have been reported on by King's College, which undertook a piece of work to evaluate the consultancy roles in 2001 (Guest et al). The themes include organisational structures, conflict issues, workload, influencing leadership, role clarity and competencies/accountability (Box 8.4).

Box 8.4   Clinical supervision themes

Organisational structures

- Role and position within the organisations
- Effect of organisational structure on patient care and management
- Leadership position and where the NTC fits in
- The lack of prepared foundation for the NTC in an organisation
- Policy changes in clinical areas
- Lack of support from the university
- Evaluation of the role's effectiveness
- Changing in organisational cultures

Conflict issues

- Resolving professional conflict
- Conflict in promoting the role
- Management of difficult processes
- Conflict with managers
- Staff conflict in the projects
- Blocks to the role
- Challenges to expert practice from professionals and how to develop strategies to respond
- Professional conflict: how to make the NTC visible and people understand the role

---

Workload

- Workload to define priorities
- Workload and the need to do everything
- Time capacity of the NTC
- Time management and time conflict
- Capacity in the role: how to say "no"
- Balancing different projects, preventing burn-out

Influencing leadership

- Ability to influence a negative attitude
- Evolving leadership
- Negative authority
- Difficulties of not managing staff and authority. the change process and how to influence it
- Modernising practice and facilitating this process
- Influencing change and generating enthusiasm
- Whether the NTC influences strategic development
- Effectiveness of the NTC role and issues of low morale

Role clarity

- Lack of clarity about role and position
- Should we be involved in research?
- How do we define our roles?
- Aspects of the NTC role and how the role has been implemented
- Conflict between the four core areas
- Recurrent insecurities about the role

Competencies/accountability

- Competencies of the NTC and how to adapt the national cancer competencies to the role
- Core competencies and conflict with the elements
- Immunisation and implications for practice and the NTC role
- Accountability and responsibility for actions
- Ownership of ideas

Activity 8.2   Feedback

The benefits of introducing clinical supervision, and how to adapt the process to your clinical area

The benefits of introducing clinical supervision can be seen from this discussion. Several points have emerged from this case study that may be useful to other NTCs:

- all NTCs require clinical supervision

- ensure that the supervisor you choose has the necessary skills to facilitate supervision successfully, whether it is individual or group supervision

- individuals have the right to choose their own supervisor rather than be allocated one by management

- it is imperative that a contract is created, agreed and signed before clinical supervision commences

- documentation of the clinical supervision session is important, and a suitable system for that nurse or clinical area must be implemented.

RECOMMENDED READING

Cody E (2003) Role models. *Nursing Management* 10(2):18–21.
Craik C, McKay AE (2003) Consultant therapists: recognising and developing expertise. *British Journal of Occupational Therapy* 66(6):281–283.
Guest D, Redfern S, Wilson-Barnett J et al (2001) *A Preliminary Evaluation of the Establishment of Nurse Midwife and Health Visitor Consultants*. Research Paper 007. Management Centre, King's College, London.
MacPhee M (2002) The role of social support networks for rural hospital nurses: supporting and sustaining the rural work force. *Journal of Advanced Nursing* 32(5):264–272.

USEFUL WEBSITES

Department of Health (2003) *Developing Key Roles for Nurses and Midwives*. HMSO, London. http://www.doh.gov.uk/newrolesfornurses/implementing.htm

REFERENCES

Bassett C (1999) *Clinical Supervision: A Guide for Implementation*. Nursing Times Books, London
Benner P (1984) From *Novice to Expert: Excellence and Power in Clinical Nursing Practice*. Addison-Wesley, California
Bird L (2002) *Action Learning Sets: The Case for Running them Online*. Work Based Learning Unit, Coventry Business School, Coventry. http://www.shef.ac.uk/nlc2002/proceedings/paper/05.htm
Bond M, Holland S (1998) *Skills of Clinical Supervision for Nurses*. Open University Press, Buckingham.
Butterworth T, Faugier J (eds) (1992) *Clinical Supervision and Mentoring in Nursing*. Chapman & Hall. London.
Chambers W and R (eds) (1990) *Chambers Dictionary*. Chambers Harrap Publishers Ltd.
Coady E (2003) Role models. *Nursing Management* 10(2):18–21.
Consultant Nurse Network (2003). http://fons.org/networks/cnn/index.htm
Craik C, McKay AE (2003) Consultant therapists: recognising and developing expertise. *British Journal of Occupational Therapy* 66(6):281–283.
Department of Health (1993) *The Evolution of Clinical Audit*. DoH, London.
Department of Health (1999) *Making a Difference: Strengthening the Nursing, Midwifery and Health Visiting Contribution to Health and Healthcare*. HMSO, London.
Gibson CH (1991) A concept analysis of empowerment. Journal of Advanced Nursing 16: 354–361.

Goodyear A (1997) The Implementation of Clinical Supervision in a NHS Trust. Unpublished MA thesis, Durham University.

Guest D, Redfern S, Wilson-Barnett J et al (2001) *A Preliminary Evaluation of the Establishment of Nurse, Midwife and Health Visitor Consultants*. Research Paper 007. Management Centre, Kings College, London.

Harker J (2001) Role of the Nurse Consultant in Tissue Viability. *Nursing Standard* 15 (49): 39–42.

Hawkins P, Shohet R (1989) *Supervision in the Helping Professions*. Open University Press, Buckingham.

Kohner N (1994) *Clinical Supervision: An Executive Summary*. King's Fund Centre, London.

Link in Nurse Consultant Site (2002). http://online.unn.ac.uk/faculties/hswe/research/PDRP/LinkNurse.htm

MacPhee M (2002) The role of social support networks for rural hospital nurses: supporting and sustaining the rural work force *Journal of Advanced Nursing* 32(5):264–272.

Manley K (2000) Consultant Nurses: refining the concept, clarifying processes and outcomes. Unpublished Doctoral Study, University of Manchester. Royal College of Nursing Institute, London.

Manley K (2001) Organisational culture and consultant nurse outcomes. I. Organisational culture. *Nursing Standard* 14(36):34–38.

McGill I, Beaty L (1995) *Action Learning: A Guide for Professional, Management and Educational Development*. Kogan Page, London.

McSherry R, Bassett C (2002) *Practice Development in the Clinical Setting: A Guide to Implementation*. Nelson Thornes Ltd, Cheltenham.

McSherry R, Kell J, Pearce P (2002) Clinical supervision and clinical governance. *Nursing Times* 98(23):30–31.

Reid B, Metclafe A (2001) Room at the top. *Health Service Journal* July 24–25.

Revans R (1979) The nature of action learning. *Management Education and Development* 10:3–23.

Rodwell CM (1996) An analysis of the concept of empowerment. Journal of Advanced Nursing 23: 305–313

Rogers C (1952*) Client Centred Therapy: Its Current Practice, Implications and Theory*. Constable, London.

Royal College of Nursing (2000) *Realising Clinical Effectiveness and Clinical Governance through Clinical Supervision*. Radcliffe Medical Press, Oxon.

United Kingdom Central Council for Nursing, Midwifery and Health Visiting (1996) Position Statement on Clinical Supervision for Nursing and Health Visiting. UKCC, London.

University of Sheffield (2003) Region's Consultant Nurses Join Forces To Benefit Patients. Press release 8 January. University of Sheffield, Sheffield.

9 Ways to Evaluate the Efficiency and Effectiveness of the Nurse/Therapist Consultant

Rob McSherry and David Mudd

INTRODUCTION

Previous chapters have defined the roles and responsibilities of the Nurse/Therapist Consultant (NTC), but means of evaluating these new roles must be developed. Much of the health and social care literature is concerned with the need for assessing and evaluating the effectiveness of professional practice.

EVALUATION: DEFINING THE TERMS

Clarke (2001) offers one definition of evaluation:

> *making a judgement about the worth or value of something. This can apply in the case of the informal subjective assessments that are part of every day life, such as when we assess the aesthetic value of a work of art. It also refers to the formal, systematic evaluations undertaken by professional evaluators or researchers.*

Activity 9.1   *Reflective question* ─────────────

The importance of evaluation in demonstrating the efficiency and effectiveness of the NTC

Write down what you think 'evaluation' means and why it is important to the future development of the NTC.

Read on and compare your findings with those in the Activity Feedback at the end of the section.

───────────────────────────────

The NTC is familiar with the language and processes associated with evaluation because they could be said to be a form of applied research with a distinctive orientation to and within practice. 'It is about undertaking a critical assessment, on as objective basis as possible, of the degree to which entire services or their component parts (e.g. diagnostic tests, treatments, caring procedures) fulfil stated goals' (St Leger et al, 1992, cited in Clarke, 2001). Debates related to evaluation are relevant to NTCs because they can provide practical advice on future developments of the role.

Cox (2000) argues that expert practice, professional leadership and research may be some of the key components required. McSherry (2004), Manley (2000a, 2000b) and Hayes and Harrison (2004) believe that the service should also look into the wider issues of the impact of the role at an organisational level as some organisations are reluctant to put evaluation into practice. The primary reasons for health and social care professionals for not engaging in the evaluation process could be said to be associated with the factors listed in Box 9.1.

Box 9.1   Obstacles preventing the development and utilisation of evaluative techniques in practice (Adapted from McSherry and Bassett, 2002. Reproduced with permission.

Selection difficulties
- How should the information be accessed?
- What is the best tool to use?
- How should the tool be implemented?
- There is difficulty in choosing an indicator tool that meets the requirements of the service.

Practice constraints
- Lack of time needed to complete and interpret the apparatus.
- The difficulty of obtaining objectivity on the part of the individuals using the measurement tools.
- The costs that can be incurred by bringing in outside agencies to perform such reviews of practice.

Interpretation/evaluation difficulties
- What to do with the data when available.
- The inability to implement the findings once the results are available.

The NTC must resolve the conditions identified in box 9.1 that are associated with the measurement and evaluation of the role. One difficulty that may arise is that an important aspect of the role is the initiation of change and how to prioritise and devise a strategy for evaluation.

PRIORITISING AND ESTABLISHING A STRATEGY FOR EVALUATION

To ensure the development of an evaluation strategy that is both efficient and effective for the needs of the NTC, the organisation and the patients, it is worth considering the advice and guidance detailed in Box 9.1, in conjunction with the following questions:

- What is meant by evaluation?
- What is the object of this evaluation?
- Why should an evaluation be carried out?
- What support/resources are there available to aid the evaluation process?
- How will the findings be shared and disseminated?

Box 9.1 suggests that there may be difficulties in selecting, applying and interpreting the evaluation as these are new posts. Some appropriate ways of assessing the role of the NTC could be undertaken in the following ways:

- *impact assessment*: This is a means of determining the impact or changes that can be attributed directly to the individual NTC within the post.
- *performance assessment*: This is a means of evaluating the wider implications of service changes and the role of the NTC within these changes.

Evaluation would seem to be an integral part of the design of new procedures in practice. It should be a key dimension contained within the business plans, job descriptions and job specifications for this post. To aid the evaluation process, however, it is clear that the rationale for evaluation must be understood. Evaluation is both a process and a product and must be seen as crucial to the NTC role. A simple yet effective way of prioritising and devising a strategy for evaluation is illustrated in Figure 9.1. This indicates that, when devising an effective strategy for evaluation, the NTC should focus on:

- types of evaluation
- a staged approach
- the key components
- objectivity and consistency.

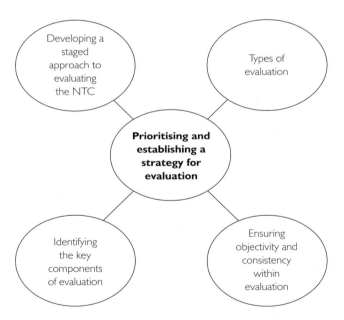

Figure 9.1   Prioritising and establishing a strategy for evaluation

Types of evaluation

The range of tasks and expectations for the NTC is wide so evaluation may seem complex. There are, however, a number of evaluation procedures already in existence that could already be adapted for the NTC (Hart and Bond, 1999). Those identified by Cheetham et al (1992), Clarke (1999), Eicok (1998) and Fairbrother (1998), for example, are for specialist practitioners but would have a use here. In addition, as an individual health and social care organisation has its own identity, it will therefore support its practitioners differently, which may add to the complexity of the task (McSherry, 2004). Furthermore, as we have already identified in previous chapters, the role, responsibilities and expectation of the NTC is often as complex and difficult to describe, as they are emergent or 'infantile positions' (Manley, 2000a; 2000b).

Stufflebeam and Shinkfield (1985) argue that 'the most important purpose of evaluation is not to prove but to improve … We cannot be sure that our goals are worthy unless we can match them to the needs of the people they are intended to serve.' It will be necessary for the NTCs evaluating the impact of the role on an established team or organisation to seek the confidence of the other professionals with whom they are working. The following practical points may help:

- seek support – you do not have to work in isolation; link with the local university or research and practice development departments
- ensure that your practice is evidence-based and current
- contribute to local and national networks
- learn from experience: by talking and sharing with others.

Activity 9.2   *Reflective question*

Ways of measuring and evaluating practices

Note down ways of measuring and evaluating the NTC role.

Read on and compare your findings with those in the Activity Feedback at the end of this section.

It may be seen from your consideration of Activity 9.2 that there is a wide variety of ways of measuring and evaluating practice. These may include clinical audit, patient satisfaction surveys, formal research studies, clinical guidelines and the utilisation of leadership and management-style assessment tools. Although we should list the merits of each approach here, it is up to practitioners to find the method best suited for their individual requirements: the NTC working with a clinical team and seeking the views of users might, for example, find a patient satisfaction survey or research focus group useful.

Three methods that the NTC could utilise are:

- audit
- comparative benchmarking
- organisational standards and accreditation.

The following section is adapted from McSherry (2002) with permission.

Audit: an ally not a threat to the NTC

Within health and social care, audit sometimes is associated with medical intervention and treatment. These clinical audits are ways of systematically measuring and improving the quality of patient care. They may be used by a single professional group or by a mixed group of health care professionals auditing the outcome of care.

To measure and evaluate new ways of working, such the NTC post, we would advocate the use of the 'multiprofessional approach to audit'. This is because many advances in or evaluations of new or existing practice(s) are based upon multiprofessional collaborations and teamworking in which it is difficult to isolate an individual's contributions to quality enhancements. Multidisciplinary audit within context of the NTC may involve:

- systematically looking at procedures used for diagnosis
- care and treatment interventions, plans or follow-ups
- examining how associated resources are used and the efficiency and effectiveness of these on the patients' outcomes
- investigating the effect of care, treatment and/or intervention on the outcome and quality of life for the patient.

The critical analysis should be used as a constructive mechanism to improve quality and demonstrate the outcome(s) for the patient, user or service. User audit can be used to support NTCs in evaluating the efficiency and effectiveness of their role and those of other colleagues' roles by focusing on issues such as:

- delivery of clinical care, treatment e.g. type of care, place of care, method of delivery
- timeliness of care/intervention e.g. appropriate time of medication, discharge planning
- outcomes of care e.g. complications, changes in function, general health perception, reduction in symptoms.

(DoH, 1993)

Multiprofessional audit is an ally to the NTC because it is about comparing our performance as an individual or team against set standards, demonstrating the effectiveness of the practice provided. This is achieved by the instigation of the audit cycle, as provided by the Department of Health (1993) and depicted in Figure 9.2, based upon observing, comparing against set standards, implementing change, setting new standards, and observing and evaluating the benefits of this to practice.

It is important that NTCs seek out the support available to aid them and/or their teams with instigating the audit process, for example, by using the Audit Department and accessing standards locally, regionally and nationally. This has been made easier over the past couple of years by the government's introduction of National Service Frameworks and National Institute for Clinical Excellence.

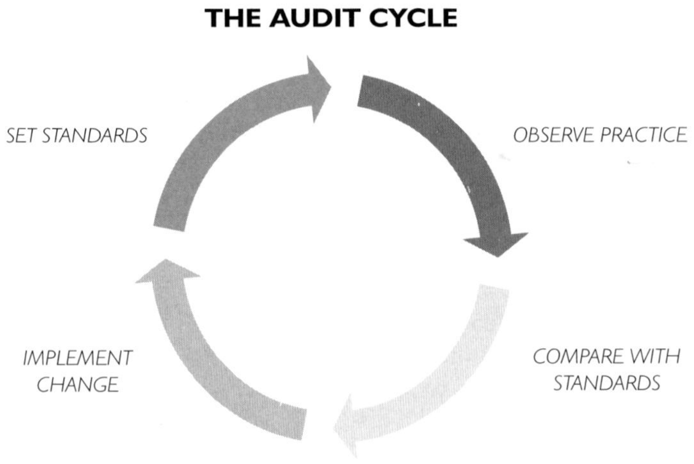

THE AUDIT CYCLE

Figure 9.2 The audit cycle adapted from the DoH (1993) The Evolution of Clinical Audit

Comparative benchmarking: promoting collaborative networking for the NTC
Kobs (1998), Ellis (1995, 1997, 2000) and Johnson (1998) discuss benchmarking as a method of improving practice. Kobs (1998) defines benchmarking as the 'continual and collaborative discipline that involves measuring and comparing the results of key processes with the best performers'. Benchmarking in this instance could be viewed as a process of promoting best practice by seeking, finding, implementing and sustaining change. It is a continuous process of measuring services and practices against other similar areas and roles (Feely, 1999, cited in McSherry and Bassett, 2002). This is a useful approach as it demonstrates the contributions that the NTC may make to teams and organisations by adopting a proactive style to measuring and evaluating new or existing practices. Benchmarking provides an opportunistic, structured approach to promoting best practice by encouraging health care professionals, teams and organisations to share and network using an identified area of care, for example comparing the levels and standards of clinical contact or education and training.

According to the works of Ellis (1995), Garry (2000), Senn (2000) and McSherry and Bassett (2002), different types of benchmarking can be undertaken depending upon the practice under review:

- *internally*, this is done by comparing similar processes but within different sections of the organisation, for example patient waiting times in different parts of outpatients
- *externally*, competitive benchmarking could be used to compare similar size organisations' performance against identified standards such as the cost of treatments or interventions
- *functional* benchmarking refers to the isolation of functional processes and compares the findings, for example, non-attendance for outpatients' appointments.

When viewed in this context, it may be argued that benchmarking may be difficult for supporting the NTC because the benchmarking process could be seen to be cumbersome and time-consuming as opposed to being an ideal mechanism for supporting and evaluating the role. However, the opposite can be said of benchmarking when transposing the principles to the NTC. Internal and external benchmarking can be used to encourage the development, evolvement and evaluation of the NTC by (Senn, 2000):

- providing a reference point for collecting information and data about the scope, purpose and remit of the post
- using real and current data associated with the post-holders to verify key roles and responsibilities
- identifying the key components that require evaluating, such as patient/clinical outcomes
- encouraging the focusing of organisational resources surrounding the post.

Put simply, the benchmarking process requires the NTC or practitioner to (Senn, 2000; Wilson, 1999):

- consider the practice requiring a benchmark
- define the process to benchmark
- select potential benchmark partners, either internally or externally
- establish data requiring capturing
- collect data from both benchmarking partners
- compare and contrast data and determine gaps in performance
- review processes for deficits
- communicate finds
- review targets for future performances
- adjust targets and develop strategy for improving practice by use of staged achievable and realistic goals
- implement changes with the involvement and endorsement of the team
- review progress after an identified period of time.

Organisational standards and accreditation: friend or foe
Over the past 15 years, the development of organisational standards and accreditation of clinical excellence have emerged as challenges and requirements for teams and organisations in demonstrating best practice against a rigorous set of criteria or standards. Initially Nursing Development Units (NDUs) (Lathlean 1997), and then Practice Development Units (PDUs) (Page et al, 1998), emerged as the forerunners for teams and organisations to utilize in demonstrating a culture based on organisational and management leadership, leadership that is founded upon a philosophy of promoting and supporting excellence in teamworking, multiprofessional collaboration or partnerships by valuing and encouraging staff to use research to advance and evaluate their practice(s).

Organisational standards and accreditation frameworks continue to emerge to assist health care professionals, teams and organisations in demonstrating an achieved level of quality for a given service. The Healthcare Commission (HC), the European Foundation for Quality Management, Investors in People (IIP), Practice/Nurse Development Unit Accreditation, Clinical Negligence Scheme for Trusts and Charter Mark to name but a few. The potential benefits of each of these frameworks lie in offering a set of criteria for measuring a given practice against a set standard or level of excellence. For example, the IIP relates to assessing organisational support and staff development, whereas the HC reviews how a health care organisation is meeting the challenge of implementing clinical governance. Both are different yet equally valuable to advancing and evaluating practice. The major disadvantages of utilizing both organisational standards and accreditation schemes within the National Health Service (NHS) is in the duplication of the time, resources and support needed for individuals, teams and organisations to collect, collate and provide the evidence to demonstrate the acquired standard(s) (McSherry et al, 2003). Health care organisations seem to be pressurised in terms of meeting not just the criteria for one award, but those for several at any one time, however, organisational standards and accreditation are essential for demonstrating acquired levels of excellence within the NHS. They provide excellent frameworks for promoting quality improvements and, as a result, support practice development.

Having critically reviewed various organisational standards and accreditation packages available for health care organisations to use, what seems to be missing that would aid practice development is a unifying and linking of these various frameworks. For example, if you go for the award of PDU/NDU and provide robust evidence to achieve the standards for valuing staff and their development, surely this evidence can be used to support similar standards within the IIP? Having reviewed the various accreditation frameworks, it would appear, according to McSherry et al (2003), that six core areas of practice have now emerged that relate to most organisational and accreditation packages within health and social care. These should also form the basis for advancing and evaluating practice(s):

1 working in organisations
2 collaborative working
3 user-focused care
4 continuous quality improvements
5 performance management
6 measuring efficiency and effectiveness.

Although the above core standards appear broad, many substandards are available to support the achievement of the standard. For example, to demonstrate working in organisations requires organisational and management support that endorses innovation via open channels of communication in encouraging and empowering staff to share ideas. Within practice development, it is about focusing individuals, teams and organisations in creating a culture in which clinical or practice excellence can occur. By focusing on the six core standards identified above, practices at an individual, team and organisational level can be measured and evaluated.

The difficulty for some NTCs may lie in becoming aware of or indeed encouraging and supporting individuals, teams and organisations in implementing such standards. We would strongly encourage NTCs to use the core standards as a possible framework for individual, team and organisational development because they offer a means and a way to ensuring consistency and objectivity of evaluating the NTC position. For more information about the newly developed **Excellence in Practice** Accreditation Scheme (EPAS) that enables comparative benchmarking to be undertaken and a level of excellence in practice to be awarded, please contact the University of Teesside Practice Development team on (01642) 342972.

Ensuring objectivity and consistency within evaluation

The difficulties and challenges facing NTCs relating to evaluating the impact of their role upon a service, individuals or organisational performance, culture or clinical outcomes, lies in devising ways and approaches that are valid, reliable and reflective of the unique situation and circumstances. Furthermore, it is important that evaluation fosters the principles of progression and support for the individual, team and the organisation. To this end, we would argue that the use of a formative and summative approaches to advancing and evaluating the position be developed. For example, formatively raising awareness of the post through the attendance of staff forums or directorate meetings, and summitively evaluating the impact of this approach through the development of formalised systems of audit. The adopting of the formative and summative approach to evaluation is useful because it provides the NTC with the opportunity to communicate, inform, engage and involve users along with a formalised framework/mechanism for measuring the effectiveness of their actions/interventions. This approach encourages consistency in the way in which evaluation is undertaken, reaffirming the need to distinguish subjective from objective data/information. The formative approach enables the subjective elements to be promoted while the summative approach reinforces the need for devising ways and methods of evaluation that are objective.

A staged approach to evaluating the NTC

There are several ways and approaches to evaluating the NTC by using either singular, or a combination of, qualitative and quantitative methods, for example surveys, interviews and focus groups. We would argue that it is essential to adopt a staged approach to evaluation. But what do we mean by a staged approach? Put simply, if you really want to demonstrate the real and realistic impact of your role and responsibilities, it is important that you and your organisation focus on devising, implementing and evaluating specific aspects of your role. For example, how do staff feel about the role? Were they consulted and informed of the role before its introduction? Table 9.1 outlines a new framework depicting how a phased approach to evaluation could be developed.

Table 9.1   A phased approach to evaluating the NTC

Stage 1: Preliminary organisational preparation/selection

Defining the key elements of the stage	Purpose	Exemplars
• Role consultation/clarification exercise	To establish clarity and purpose/scope remit of the post, and to identify/confirm source of funding	Staff consultation groups/forums
• Pre selection	Ensuring that the job description and personal specification are robustly developed and meet the needs of users and the service	Sharing the key aspects of the role and seeking/auditing users' perceptions and attitudes
• Interview	Important to ensure that the correct person is appointed for the post and meets the requirements of the users/service	Robust interview and selection criteria; presentation that incorporates a diverse range of stakeholders
• Post interview	Conforming to the parameters, scope and remit of the post	Consultation with users and professional groups to communicate role relationships

Stage 2: Commencing/getting started

• Induction and settling-in period	Imperative to ensure that the NTC meets and greets users associated with the service to build working relationships and confidence in the individual and organisation	Provide forums for work-based induction to the role of the NTC supported by informative literature
• Getting to know the **role**: scope, purpose, remit of the post	Undertake individual supervision and specific role analysis to identify the immediate, short- and long-term priorities for the post. This should be undertaken in conjunction with organisational objectives, personal development reviews and action-planning processes	A systematic approach should be adopted, taking into account individual and organisational needs/priorities so that the best start can be offered. A solid foundation from the outset will ensure that the role is implemented and evaluated effectively. The role analysis can be used as a benchmark for evaluating performance and outcomes later
	A robust action plan with time scales associated with how the various component parts are to be performed and evaluated should be produced	The utilising of self-assessment templates and personal development reviews/action plans provides focused direction and a framework for evaluation

• Resources and support	A review of individual and organisational needs and resource issues should have been undertaken with the post-holder and employer to ensure that they have sufficient support and resources	NTCs should have adequate support and resources to meet their needs and priorities. These should be part of the business case/planning process
• Network and sharing	Fundamental to raising awareness of the post and in seeking support to undertake the role	The development of and attendance at local, regional and national NTC networks is imperative to the furtherance of the individual, organisation and profession

Stage 3: Midpoint (implementation) evaluation

– Deciphering and actioning the scope, purpose and remit of the post	Important to review whether the priorities and the development of the systems/processes associated with implementing the key aspects of stage 2 have been introduced	To establish a series of audits to see whether individual users and the organisation are aware of the role and its priorities

Stage 4: Performance/outcome evaluation

– Formal internal and external independent evaluation	The most fundamental aspect of the evaluation process in trying to draw together the overall impact of the role on performance and outcome, both internally and externally	This aspect of evaluation should hopefully have been thought through in the developmental stage. If, however, it was not, it is about seeking the support and guidance to evaluate the overall impact of the role. Some organisations may choose to do this independently or in conjunction with the post-holders and an independent organisation. What is important is that this formal evaluation occurs

According to Table 9.1, it can be seen that a phased approach could be developed to support the evaluation of the NTC in the future. The limitation of the framework is that it does not provide all the detail of what and when to evaluate. We would argue that this is the responsibility of individuals and the organisation.

Stage 1 (Preliminary organisational preparation/selection) should provide extensive information about the essential characteristics of the NTC post, its purpose, scope and remit demonstrable through extensive organisational and service planning and consultation culminating in the merger of a:

- robust business case/plan
- identified funding stream
- job description
- personal specification
- interview selection process and criteria
- appointed specification plan
- template for induction.

An evaluation of this stage would focus on issues such as the efficiency and effectiveness of the organisation in consulting and communicating about the post and its scope and remit during the pre–post interview and appointment period. This is imperative in ensuring that the right person has been appointed for the right post at the right time.

Stage 2 (Commencing/getting started) is, for several reasons, an important stage in ensuring the evaluation of the NTC. First, this stage provides the time and opportunity for the NTC to engage with and meet users/stakeholders to tell them about the way in which the role and responsibilities could be delivered and evaluated. Second, it is about reviewing the purpose, scope and remit of the post in an operational form and identifying the necessary support and resources to meet these needs. Third, this stage should culminate with the development of a role analysis, action plan and maybe an operational/strategic implementation plan or policy highlighting how and why you have prioritised what you have. In essence, this stage breaks the job description and specification plan down into manageable sections and how these will be realised with the organisation, for example deciding how much of your role will be devoted to the clinical or research components of the role. Fourth, it is worth investing a good deal of time at this stage because these priorities, goals and actions could arguably form the basis of an independent evaluation once the role has been established.

An evaluation of this stage should focus on issues such as:

- undertaking a role analysis to prioritise key aims/objectives
- the development of action or personal development plans
- resources and support review
- an implementation strategy for the role, outlining specific activities and how these will be monitored and evaluated
- the development of individual and organisation networks
- identification of the mechanisms for sharing and disseminating the evolvement of the role.

If stage two is rigorously and robustly invested and implemented, the impact on stage 3 will be evident.

Stage 3 (Midpoint (implementation) evaluation) should be undertaken at around 6–12 months after commencing the post. The inclusion of a midpoint evaluation is fundamental for several reasons. First, it enables you to review the systems and processes that you have put in place for achieving the role and your priorities highlighted in stage 1. Second, it enables you to change direction or approaches if things are not going the way you anticipated. Third, it provides a good opportunity to share and disseminate progress to date and seek confirmation from peers/colleagues and users about what they feel and think about the progress of the role so far. Fourth, the findings from such an evaluation can be used to see whether the original purpose, scope and remit of the post are what is emerging or whether amendments may need to be made. Finally, it is about learning and reflecting from experience and using this to build your confidence in the post and the furtherance of the post. Remember, at this stage it is not about failure!

An evaluation of this stage should focus on issues such as:

- seeking views and opinions from stakeholders/users regarding role expectation and activities
- communication infrastructures
- personal and role characteristics/attributes
- acceptations/recognition of the role
- the effectiveness of engagement and involvement with the role
- feedback on the role analysis/aims/objectives and priorities
- credibility within the role
- role boundary and management.

If you are efficient and effective in implementing and evaluating key activities in stage 3, you can feel comfortable in knowing that the role is heading in the right direction and you can begin to put the more formal or summative systems in place for stage 4.

Stage 4 (Performance/outcome evaluation) is by far the most important stage of evaluating the NTC, for several reasons. First, it enables a thorough review to be undertaken of how efficient and effective the purpose, scope and remit of the post have been in doing what they were supposed to do. Second, utilising this extensive evaluation focuses on demonstrating the impact of the role in relation to individual and organisational performances against set standards such as the National Service Framework, or in promoting modernisation of the NHS through introducing new and innovative ways of working or changing existing practices or service provision. Third, the utilisation of independent evaluation by engaging independent internal and/or external parties enables an evaluation to be undertaken that will encourage the post-holder to progress or change practices for the furtherance of themselves and others. Fourth, although an independent review/evaluation is daunting and could possibly be perceived to be anxiety- and stress-provoking, the approach fits nicely with the HC's techniques for reviewing, adding strength to the findings. Finally, the formal independent review enables a whole-systems approach to evaluation to be undertaken, focusing on the impact of the role on structures, processes and outcomes (McSherry 2004). An evaluation of this stage should focus on issues such as:

* role implementation/achievement
* enhanced quality and patient outcomes
* cost-effectiveness through organisational development
* user satisfaction
* career progression
* recruitment and retention
* sharing and dissemination
* networks and relationship building
* consultancy.

In brief, this staged approach to evaluation provides a new developmental framework for NTCs and/or organisations to use and apply in developing systems and processes to evaluate the efficiency and effectiveness of their role. The future of the NTC undoubtedly depends on the sharing and dissemination of findings from using different approaches to evaluation to elicit information specific to their unique role.

Evaluation: its importance to the future of the NTC

It was recommend by Guest et al (2001) that 'there is a strong case for using these varied experiences to provide a set of guidelines for all sponsors and nursing directors to ensure that initial entry into the role and early socialisation is as effective as possible'. The staged approach to evaluation provides individuals and organisations with an opportunistic framework for meeting the recommendations made by Guest et al (2001). The future of the NTC depends on their meeting the challenges of organisational demands, cultural differences and changes in clinical practice. These positions should be regarded as collaboration between the NTC and professional groups, in which working together 'could lead to the development of progressive healthcare, which will ultimately benefit patients' (Jones, 2002). The realisation of the NTC posts lies in seeking out and reviewing what people think and feel, as is eloquently depicted in Case Study 9.1, A stakeholder approach to evaluating the NTC (below).

CONCLUSION

Evaluation is undoubtedly a complex procedure, and processes will need to be put in place to measure the impact of the NTC role on both individual and organisation. Evaluation, within the context of this chapter, is (Clarke, 2001):

> not only about measuring the effectiveness of particular interventions by focusing on health outcomes but is also about illuminating the process going on in nursing [therapist] care. While outcomes are often best measured by quantitative indicators, process issues are more amenable to qualitative analysis.

SUMMARY OF KEY POINTS

- Evaluation is relevant to the NTC because it focuses on the subjective and objective aspects associated with measuring the efficiency and effectiveness of a role or service.
- Evaluation is strongly recognised and regarded in contemporary health and social care literature for demonstrating the efficiency and effectiveness of an intervention, treatment action or decision in care.
- Several types and ways for evaluating the NTC role are already in existence that could be modified or adapted to suit the needs of the NTC.
- It is important that evaluation fosters the principles of progression and support for the individual, team and organisation. To this end, we would argue that a formative and summative approach to advancing and evaluating the position should be used.
- A staged approach to evaluation is fundamental.
- NTCs needs to adopt a creative and flexible approach using a variety of internal and external methods, departments and resources to demonstrate their efficiency and effectiveness in practice.

Activity 9.1   *Feedback* _____

The importance of evaluation in demonstrating the efficiency and effectiveness of the NTC

Evaluation should be viewed and regarded as an integral aspect of the NTC post and not as an adjunct to the role. Evaluation should start not when the NTC comes into the post but when the post is identified and developed. Evaluation must be supported and resourced, which is why it is important to reflect this in the business case, job/personal specification and job description. Evaluation is not easy, but it is fundamentally important for the NTC, the team and the organisation.

CASE STUDY 9.1   A STAKEHOLDER APPROACH TO EVALUATING THE NTC

Aidan Mullan, Rob McSherry and Dave Mudd

The past 10 years have seen considerable development in the number and function of advanced nursing roles, such as Lecturer Practitioners and, in the past four years, Nurse Consultants. However, many ambiguities exist about the nature and value of such roles. The literature on advanced roles tends to focus on variations in the definition and nature of the role (see, for example, Eicock, 1998; Fairbrother, 1998), with considerable discussion on the lack of consensus that exists in clinical practice on the current nature of the role. There is a paucity of studies attempting to evaluate the role, existing evidence being based on small-scale studies evaluating the introduction of advanced nursing roles (e.g. McGee, 1998; Murphy, 2000). A recent national quantitative evaluative study into nursing roles failed to provide data on the lived experience of Nurse Consultants and relationships with other health professionals (Guest et al, 2001). There does not appear to be any consideration of possible future development of the role.

Considerable investment in these roles has, however, been made on both a local and a national scale. There is a need to identify the value of the investment in these posts, particularly the benefits to health care activity. Furthermore, policy decisions indicate that the posts will remain for some time. Unfortunately, there is limited information that could be used to inform future developments of the role.

Methodology

One of the limitations of traditional approaches to evaluation of a role or service is the assumption that it is possible to achieve consensus about the nature of any evaluation strategy (Cheetham et al, 1992). Achieving consensus can, however, be problematic when interested parties have unique sets of interests. Smith and Cantley (1985) believe that it is possible to overcome the problem of absent consensus, but instead involve stakeholders in the conduct of an evaluation. In specific terms, stakeholders are consulted on the nature of evaluation questions, the sample, definitions of successful outcomes and the measurement of effectiveness of an activity (Fink, 1993).

The rationale behind this approach is the belief that stakeholder participation offers a wide range of interested parties the opportunity to influence policy decisions and allows a range of perspectives to be used to inform the collection and interpretation of findings, as well as promoting utilisation of the findings (Shaw, 1999). Ovretveit (1998) describes a number of features of stakeholder evaluation that include the identification of main stakeholders with an interest in the evaluation plus understanding and describing the interpretations that different parties make of events. In addition, a final step in the evaluation involves assessing the extent to which the evaluation's conclusions meet stakeholders' criteria for 'success' (Cheetham et al, 1992).

This evaluation will follow the principles of stakeholder evaluation in using a collaborative approach by allowing key parties to participate in the design, conduct and interpretation of the evaluation. In this evaluation, the key participants have been identified as the Nurse Consultants and line managers. The nature of the resources available precludes the involvement of additional stakeholders.

Methods

Each Nurse Consultant was allocated a member of the project team as the interviewer. This person was responsible for obtaining the sample, the data and the initial data analysis for the individual Nurse Consultant.

Sample
The study was based around the three Nurse Consultants currently at the University Hospital of Hartlepool at this first stage of the evaluation. A collaborative purposive

sampling technique was used. Discussions involved each Nurse Consultant, the principal investigator, their allocated researcher, the Director of Nursing or nominated deputy and the line manager, who identified up to 10 participants (excluding service users in this stage of the evaluation), who were able to provide detailed, objective and relevant information to inform the aims of the evaluation in all of the facets of the Nurse Consultant role. This meant that the total evaluation sample consisted of 30 participants (as well as the three Nurse Consultants themselves).

If two or more different Nurse Consultants nominated the same person, that person had the option to provide data in relation to either one, both or neither of the Nurse Consultants. Furthermore, the nature of the sample identified by each individual Nurse Consultant was discussed and agreed with the individual's line manager, the clinical lead for the speciality, the Director of Nursing (or nominated deputy) and the principal investigator. If any disagreements arose, negotiations took place with the project team to finalise the nature of the sample.

Data collection

Data were collected using individual semi-structured interviews. The agenda for the interviews was developed by the project team through a thematic analysis of topics for possible discussion suggested by each Nurse Consultant in conjunction with their line manager. A broad semi-structure was agreed in preparation for interviewing the other health professionals and guided rather than defined the nature of the interview:

- What were your expectations of the role of the Nurse Consultant?
- In what way has the individual fulfilled the role of the Nurse Consultant?
- What aspects of the work of the Nurse Consultant do you value most? Why?
- In what way does the Nurse Consultant fit into the team?
- What aspects of the Nurse Consultant role would you like the individual to work more on?
- In what way is work better since the Nurse Consultant came into post?

Data analysis

The data collected in relation to each Nurse Consultant were analysed following the principles of thematic analysis, as described by Bowling (1997). The allocated member of the project team produced a draft report that was discussed with the Nurse Consultant to promote validity in analysis of the relevant data. The project team then undertook a preliminary analysis of all individual reports with the aim of producing a draft project report that would reflect the findings of the various individual reports. After that, project members produced individual reports that the project team integrated to produce the draft project report, which was then discussed at a conference involving all participants and the project team. The purpose of this conference was to promote both the validity and the acceptability of findings, as well as generating possible developments in the Nurse Consultant role.

Preliminary emerging results

The Nurse Consultant is undoubtedly a significant role and contributes to the modernisation of the NHS, the future career pathways and the professional imagery of nursing. The preliminary results of this evaluative study identify the practical issues, concerns and realities of the posts. A combination of individual and organisational factors has the potential to influence these posts.

Recommendations

- That a phased approach to establishing, implementing and evaluating the NTC role is adopted.
- That awareness of the value of the NTC post is raised.
- That NTCs must be appropriately resourced and supported.

Activity 9.2   *Feedback*

Ways of measuring and evaluating practices

Evaluation is a complex yet integral aspect of the NTC role. The NTC should remember that there are already in existence several approaches to evaluate the role for its efficiency and effectiveness; audit, benchmarking, formal research and accreditation to name but a few. The key to successful evaluation is in using the most appropriate method(s) to suit your particular circumstance.

RECOMMENDED READING

Hayes J, Harrison A (2004) Consultant nurses in mental health: a discussion of the historical and policy context of the role. *Journal of Psychiatric and Mental Health Nursing* 11:185–188.

McSherry R, Bassett C (eds) (2002) *Practice Development in the Clinical Setting: A Guide to Implementation*. Nelson Thornes Ltd, Cheltenham.

REFERENCES

Bowling A (1997) *Research Methods in Health*. Open University Press, Buckingham.

Cheetham J, Fuller R, Mclvor G, Fetch A (1992) *Evaluating Social Work Effectiveness*. Open University Press, Buckingham.

Clarke A (1999) *Evaluation Research*. Sage. London.

Clarke A (2001) Evaluation research in nursing and health care. *Nurse Researcher* 8(3):4–14.

Cox CL (2000) The nurse consultant: an advanced practitioner? *Nursing Times* 96: 13, 48.

Department of Health (1993) *The Evolution of Clinical Audit*. DoH, London.

Eicock K (1998) Lecturer practitioner: a concept analysis. *Journal of Advanced Nursing* 28(5):1092–1098.

Ellis J (1995) Using benchmarking to improve practice *Nursing Standard* 9(35):25–28.

Ellis J (1997) Paediatric benchmarking: a review of its development. *Nursing Standard* 12, 2, 43–46.

Ellis J (2000) Making a difference to practice: clinical benchmarking. II. *Nursing Standard* 14(33):32–35.

Fairbrother P (1998) Lecturer practitioners: a literature review. *Journal of Advanced Nursing* 27(2):274–279.

Fink A (1993) *Evaluating Fundamentals: Guiding Health Programs, Research and Policy*. Sage, Newbury Park.

Garry R (2000) Benchmarking: A Prescription for Healthcare. *Journal Nursing Administrator* (JNursAdm) 30, 9, 397–398.

Guest D, Redfern S, Wilson-Barnet J et al (2001) A Preliminary Evaluation of the Establishment of Nurse, Midwife and Health Visitor Consultants. *Research Paper 007. Mangement Centre, Kings College, London.*

Hart E, Bond M (1999) *Action Research for Health and Social Care: A Guide to Practice*. Open University Press, Buckingham.

Johnson JN (1998) Making self-regulation credible through benchmarking, peer review, appraisal – and management. Editorials *BMJ* 316–1847–1848.

Jones P (2002) Consultant nurses and their potential impact upon health care delivery. *Clinical Medicine* 2, 139–40.

Kobs EJA (1998) Getting started on benchmarking. *Outcomes in Management and Nursing Practice* 2(1):45–48.

Lathlean J, Vaugh B (1997) *Directory of NDU Activities*. Kings Fund, London.

Manley K (2000a) Organisational culture and nurse consultant outcomes. II. Nurse outcomes. *Nursing Standard* 14(37):34–38.

Manley K (2000b) Organisational culture and nurse consultant outcomes. I. Organisational culture. *Nursing Standard* 14(36):34–38.

McGee P (1998) An evaluation of the lecturer-practitioner role in the independent health care sector. Journal of Clinical Nursing 7, 3 251–256.

McSherry R, Bassett C (eds) (2002) *Practice Development in the Clinical Setting: A Guide to Implementation*. Nelson Thornes Ltd, Cheltenham.

McSherry R, Kell J, Mudd D (2003) Practice development: best practice using Excellence in Practice Accreditation Scheme. *British Journal of Nursing* 12(10):623–629.

McSherry R (2004) Practice development and health care governance: a recipe for modernisation. *Journal of Nursing Management* 12:137–146.

Murphy M (2000) Collaborating with practitioners in teaching and research a model for developing the role of the nurse lecturer in practice areas. JAN 31, 3 704–714.

Ovretveit J (1998) *Evaluating Health Interventions*. Open University Press, Buckingham.

Page S, Allsop D, Casley S (1998) *The Practice Development Unit: An Experiment in Multidisciplinary Innovation*. Whurr, London.

St Leger AS (1992) *Evaluating Health Services' Effectiveness*. Open University Press, Buckingham.

Senn FG (2000) Benchmarking: your performance measurement and improvement tool. *Gastroenterology Nursing* 23(5):221–225.

Smith G and Cantley C (1985) *Assessing Healthcare: A study in organisational evaluation*. Open University, Milton Keynes.

Stufflebeam DL, Shinkfield AJ (1985) *Systematic Evaluation: A Self-Instrumental Guide to Theory and Practice*. Kluwer Nijhoff, Dordrecht.

Wilson M (1999) Using Benchmarking Practices for the Learning Resources Center. *Nurse Educator* 24, 4, 16–20.

10 CONCLUSION: THE WAY AHEAD

Sarah Johnson

THE WAY AHEAD FOR THE NURSE/THERAPIST CONSULTANT

The NHS Plan (DoH, 1999a) has laid the foundations for the redesign and restructuring of health care in the United Kingdom. The implementation of this through *Making a Difference* (DoH, 1999b) and *Meeting the Challenge* (DoH, 2000) has led to significant changes and the development of exciting new posts. The Nurse/Therapist Consultant (NTC) has, as one of these posts, certainly broken new ground for both the service and the post-holders. The first generation of NTCs has now been in post for about five years, and allied health professional (AHP) Consultants for two. At a recent conference, 'Seize the Day', at Wakefield in July 2004, Kay East, the AHP Lead at the Department of Health, raised the issue of sustainability of these posts in the changing workplace.

Cusack (2004) reports on a survey of AHP Consultants conducted by Jackie Turnpenny at the Modernisation Agency Leadership Centre between May and July 2003. Some described the first impressions of their new roles and responsibilities of the posts as:

- 'scary'
- 'an exciting opportunity with freedom to set own goals and plans'
- 'daunting as no role model to follow'
- 'it felt good, I felt I had been recognised for the responsibility and hard work undertaken daily'.

These AHP pioneers were, like the nurses before them, challenged as they established this new role within the workplace. As the posts are few in number, it can be an isolatory experience as the NTC may no longer feel part of the local professional management team or part of the local higher education team. Bent (2004) suggests that networking with other NTCs and keeping up to date with published research are important.

The issues in Table 10.1 have been identified and should be considered when planning for the development of the NTC.

Table 10.1 Planning for the future

Identified issues	Development needs	Action to be taken
Development of posts	Strategic rather than local development Management support across Acute and Primary Care Trusts	Strategic Health Authorities to take lead Political lobbying for posts Through workforce planning in locality Implementation of *Agenda for Change* (DoH, 2003)

Staff development	Moving from Specialist to Consultant Identifying development needs within the post	Clinical and academic development opportunities Through appraisal and personal reflection
Support in post	Often work in isolation New posts	Develop support networks Mentorship
Research and development	Need to initiate research projects in practice	Develop links with local higher education institutions
Education programmes	Developing continued professional development programmes in practice	Develop courses and pathways that link theory and practice

Development of posts

These posts were, until now, often developed in an ad hoc way across the country. Current NTCs may have worked with managers to argue and evidence the case for such a post in service, and it appears that many have been developed with the government's waiting list targets as the key focus. In physiotherapy, for example (the largest group among the AHPs), musculoskeletal therapists predominate, as this area of practice can, with appropriate staffing, quite quickly tackle the current waiting list initiatives. Similarly, some of the Consultant posts within nursing have centred on tackling issues identified in National Services Frameworks such as that for coronary artery disease.

Now that the Strategic Health Authorities (SHAs) are taking on the development of posts, a wider perspective can be taken, which should help both the identification of need and the allocation of funding to these posts. Initially, no new funding came with these posts, and they have had to be created largely from underspend and vacancies; this short-term answer will not, however, guarantee the sustainability of posts.

The Chartered Society of Physiotherapists, led by Richard Griffin, is lobbying Parliament to encourage more positive action and designated funding for the development of posts. The original target of, for example, 250 for AHPs by 2004 seems a distant memory as those currently (July 2004) in post number 41, with a small number more in the development stage.

The Agenda for Change (DoH 2003) will identify a route through to Consultant (Band 8). There are four levels (a, b, c, d) within this band, and it is very likely that a 'gateway' from Specialist Practitioner to Consultant will be identified at level 'c' in order that the seniority of this post is evident. The posts are different in focus, which will have to be defined in personal specifications and job descriptions, as discussed earlier in this book.

Staff development

Medicine has a clearly defined and acknowledged route to Consultant that is accepted by both the professions and the public This, however, has not yet developed for NTC posts, which has meant that post-holders come with a range of experience and qualifications. Once in post, individual NTCs should, through appraisal, have identified specific learning needs and development. At this level, it seems appropriate for newly appointed NTCs to be paired with a 'buddy' – an experienced NTC who will be able to guide the newcomer to appropriate training and development opportunities.

The professional bodies, for example the College of Occupational Therapists and the Chartered Society of Physiotherapists, have identified job specifications and job descriptions for the posts, but there is no current staff development that will clearly lead a practitioner to Consultant level. This involves extended professional practice alongside a Doctorate in practice. The move from Specialist to Consultant is where staff development needs to be focused, and this can be through a range of routes. This is where the universities will play a key role, as they can work with clinical colleagues in developing practice-based programmes to promote higher-level thinking and research skills. This will ensure that new services are evidence-based. Master's programmes that enable students to base their assignments within their workplace will be of real value and will help move both individual and practice on in the way envisaged in the modernisation literature. Clinical Doctorates and Professional Doctorates will enable students to develop their academic knowledge and skills further by examining and evaluating their practice in greater depth and implementing practice-based research. New programmes, such as the one currently being developed by the author and Fleur Kitsell at the Wessex Deanery, Southampton University, will help AHPs prepare for Consultant posts.

Support in post

These posts are, by their very design, often isolated, and the NTC may be physically many miles away from another at the same level. For example, in the south west of England, there is currently only one AHP Consultant between Bristol and Land's End and fewer than five NTCs for the region. This makes supportive networks difficult to implement. Nurses have developed networks that follow the National Service Frameworks – there is, for example, one for Older People and one for Emergency Care. These individuals have high-level influence and meet regularly with the Secretary of State for Health, therefore having direct links to developing policy. The AHPs have one network, which has been initiated by the Leadership Centre and meets monthly in London. This, however, will cease to exist from April 2005 as the modernisation agency is devolved to the regions.

It is envisaged that local networks, such as the one for occupational therapists (Oliveck, 2004), will develop as numbers grow. Networks may be virtual, as with the nursing one based at the University of Northumbria. The Internet can support a number of exciting channels for communication, ranging from electronic journals and discussion forums to bringing people together through satellite video-conferencing. As technology improves, this could become a very clear route for those separated by distance to feel supported in the workplace.

Mentorship has long being recognised in nursing and higher education as a way of supporting new staff in post. It is particularly helpful where the nature of the post is different or new to the post-holder and the roles and responsibilities may appear daunting and overwhelming. The first two years in post appear to be the most challenging as NTCs carve out a new role and develop their post. The first generation of NTCs could develop this model as a way of supporting and encouraging future consultants into post.

Organising conferences and study days and carrying out joint research projects are methods that help bring like-minded individuals together and create the support that may be missing on a day-to-day basis; this may be a route forward for some.

Research and development

One of the key roles of these posts is research and practice development. Future NTCs may have or will be working towards Master's degrees or Doctorates. In order that these are appropriate to practice, NTCs should become involved in joint writing groups with academic colleagues to plan and write appropriate programmes for those wanting to become Consultants and for those in post. Joint teaching posts, such as Lecturer/Practitioner posts, help to build links between theory and practice. NTCs are beginning to take on this role, feeding into specialist practice modules within Master's programmes and undertaking research projects with academic colleagues.

Universities are centres of excellence for research; the design, funding and implementation of research projects are their business, and NTCs should not be diffident in approaching their academic colleagues in their field for advice and guidance. Working together will truly bring evidence-based practice to the workplace and help raise standards of care for patients.

NTCs may need to develop continued professional development (CPD) programmes for staff in practice. These days, the universities that run preregistration education programmes for health and social care often have a wide programme of CPD funded by the Workforce Development Confederation. If the NTC wishes to develop training for practice, it often will be possible to organise the learning into a module or short programme that can carry academic credits – this will then enable individuals to gain both academic and clinical credibility for their study and may lead them on in their future development. This thinking fits well with Agenda for Change (DoH, 2004) as staff will be able to identify learning through their annual appraisal and then link this to the Knowledge and Skills Framework – leading them up the 'skills escalator'.

CONCLUSION

These are the posts that the professions have been waiting for, and the opportunities should not be wasted. They are new, they are ground-breaking, and they are difficult. In order for the modernisation agenda to be fully realised, it is important that these posts succeed, as these new clinical leaders are an important part of the modernisation agenda.

REFERENCES

Bent J (2004) How effective and valued are nurse consultants in the UK? *Nursing Times* 100(25):34–36.

Cusack L (2004) The Consultant AHP. *OT News* 12(2):19.

Department of Health (1999a) *The NHS Plan. A Plan for Investment. A Plan for Reform.* HMSO, London.

Department of Health (1999b) *Making a Difference: Strengthening the Nursing, Midwifery and Health Visiting Contribution to Health and Healthcare.* HMSO, London.

Department of Health (2000) *Meeting the Challenge.* HMSO, London.

Department of Health (2003) *Agenda for Change.* HMSO, London.

Oliveck M (2004) Consulting the consultants. *OT News* 12(2):18–19.

INDEX

Page references in *italics* indicate figures and those in **bold** tables or boxes.